THE DYCZYNSKI PROGRAM

THE DYCZYNSKI PROGRAM

HEALING
THE INTELLIGENT HEART

Jerzy Dyczynski

dyczynskitelehealth.co

CONTENTS

You should seek advice from a qualified healthcare professional

Information in this book is intended as general summary information that is made available to the public. It is not intended to provide specific medical advice, or to take the place of a qualified healthcare professional. Information resources are designed to help readers to better understand their own health and diagnosed conditions. You are urged to consult with qualified health care providers for diagnosis and treatment and for answers to personal health care questions.

For Angela and Fatima

One

About Dr Dyczynski

Dr Jerzy Dyczynski MD, MBA is a medical doctor who is passionate about both mainstream and holistic medicine. He has worked as a medical doctor and a medical acupuncturist for more than 30 years in Poland, Germany, Switzerland and Australia, in public and private health care systems.

Jerzy is a cardiologist, an internal medicine specialist and a Doctor of Medical Sciences. He has published papers in over 70 international journals and has given more than a hundred scientific presentations on the global stage. He completed studies as an acupuncturist in Beijing from 1991 to 1997.

Dr Jerzy attained qualifications in medical quality management for physicians of the Bavarian Medical Council, Munich, between 1999 and 2000, including training: moderation, medical leadership, epidemiology, information systems, organizational techniques, quality dimensions and methods of interdisciplinary safety models, in business process management, quality management strategies, and quality and risk management.

Dr Jerzy received his doctorate in Cardiology in 2002 and graduated with a medical MBA in the management of outpatient and integrated medical care.

Since 2007 he has lived in Perth, Western Australia, where he has practiced as a rural GP and as a postgraduate researcher in heart-brain medicine. He has practiced as an acupuncturist at Edith Cowan University, as well as in private practice in Western Australia.

Jerzy has practiced Qi-gong and Kung Fu for more than 20 years and has published two books on the nexus between Eastern and Western medicine.

The Dyczynski Program
Healing the Intelligent Heart
https://dyczynskitelehealth.co/

Eli King Press, PO Box 556, Nedlands 6009 Western Australia

Jerzy Dyczynski

You should seek advice from a qualified healthcare professional

Information in this book is intended as general summary information that is made available to the public. It is not intended to provide specific medical advice, or to take the place of a qualified healthcare professional. Information resources are designed to help readers to better understand their own health and diagnosed conditions. You are urged to consult with qualified health care providers for diagnosis and treatment and for answers to personal health care questions.

Table of Contents

Introduction

Heart disease remains the number one cause of death around the world, even in the era of the Covid-19 pandemic. Our biological factors (immune response) and general behaviour (habits) can strongly determine the consequences of COVID-19.

Most of those who die of COVID-19 have pre-existing conditions, including hypertension, diabetes mellitus, and cardiovascular disease. According to 2020 March data from the United States, 89% of those hospitalised with Covid-19 had pre-existing conditions.

The Italian Istituto Superiore di Sanità reported in 2020 that, out of 8.8% of deaths where medical charts were available, 96.1% of people had at least one comorbidity (pre-existing condition) with the average person having 3.4 diseases. The most common pre-existing conditions were hypertension (66% of deaths), ischemic heart disease (27.6% of deaths), and atrial fibrillation (23.1% of deaths) https://en.wikipedia.org/wiki/COVID-19

Every day brings new, disturbing statistics that chart the havoc wrought by heart disease:

1. Health data brought together from more than 190 countries show heart disease remains the No. 1 global cause of death with 17.3 million deaths each year, according to "Heart Disease and Stroke Statistics — 2015 Update: A Report From the American Heart Association

2. Another 17 million people worldwide are now tragically losing their lives through the sudden cardiac death (SCD) every year. This condition is also striking so-called "healthy people," who have no previous symptoms of heart disease prior to their sudden cardiac death

3. Sixty million Americans suffer from cardiovascular disease and one person dies every 30 seconds from heart disease

4. Every single day, 80,000 people worldwide suffer a heart attack; 30 million suffer heart attacks in one year

5. Heart disease is the leading cause of death in American and Australian women. It affects one out of every two females in the United States

6. Each year, 2.5 million women in United States are hospitalized for cardiac disorders and about 500,000 die because of them

7. More women are dying from heart-related disease than from breast, lung, uterine, and ovarian cancer combined

8. Heart disease does not just kill the elderly , it is the leading cause of death for all Americans age 35 and older and is the leading

cause of death in both men and women, and among all racial and ethnic groups

9. Premature deaths in alarming numbers are occurring in young people, including students and well-trained athletes, who are neither overweight nor considered to have risk factors.

As these statistics show, an increasing number of people are struck down by heart disease. It appears that the heart has lost the battle, or failed to fulfil the complex and perfect task of beating for a long and healthy life. This loss of life is not only a failure of the heart. Our brain is affected too by the hibernating heart. The brain enters hibernation following the heart's dysfunctional state. It could be just long enough to result in a confused state of mind or even to produce a mini stroke.

The number of invasive cardiac procedures performed is increasing. In 2018, in the USA, 965,000 of angioplasties with a stent implantation were performed. This number is enormous. In Asia, more than 600,000 coronary angiographies to open a blocked coronary vessel with a catheter balloon were necessary. In Europe, more than 750,000 people underwent such interventions with a stent implantation. All these procedure are invasive. They carry a significant risk of adverse reactions, including death, during the procedure. Studies have demonstrated a risk of 2% for all patients undergoing invasive opening of a coronary artery blockage.

* * *

In a lifetime of 80 years, the human heart beats about 4 billion times. But in too many cases it beats much less.

The heart is the key to human health and wellbeing.

We're inclined to think of the heart as just a pump, the thing that pushes blood around your body. And although pumping blood is an important function of the heart, it's by no means the only one.

Recent research has shown that, far from being just a pump, the human heart is second only to the brain in its cognitive activity. While the brain is instrumental in controlling much of what the heart does, the awareness of the heart in turn drives a vast number of bodily functions and directly regulates human health. Your heart is packed with neurons, just like your brain and central nervous system. It has a profound intelligence that is only now becoming understood.

The discovery of the heart's intelligence is a game-changer. It heralds a major shift in the perception of healing. We are standing at the frontier of modern heart science and looking at an exciting, futuristic landscape.

A new evidence-based, holistic model is emerging. This new, cardio-centred model is changing the field of holistic heart health and medical physics. The accelerating pace of change in medical science and the expansion of medical physics represent a new dawn of human health and wellbeing.

A New World of Knowledge at Our Fingertips

Medical science is advancing rapidly, faster than ever. Global communication networks expand faster, further and deeper, producing an explosion of data. We're living in an age of information, and human destiny is being shaped by this. What happens to humanity in general, and quite specifically what will happen to us individually, will be determined in large part by the vast sweep of modern communications and information technology. Researchers are able to learn from and exchange ideas with colleagues all around the world in real time. A breakthrough that occurs in Rabat on Monday will affect the way research is conducted on seven continents on Tuesday. Our connectivity and access to a growing universe of knowledge drives an accelerating wave of discovery and development, which in turn gives rise to new cures, treatments and understanding.

New, advanced fields of medical knowledge have developed, with multi-dimensional possibilities holding out the promise of perfect, holistic health. New opportunities of precision medicine based on artificial intelligence are waiting for every person interested in pursuing a healthy lifestyle.

But the importance of this new age of information isn't limited to the world of scientific research. Now it's personal. Now everybody has easy access to cutting-edge global knowledge and exponential growing wisdom. You can incorporate and apply this knowledge yourself directly to daily decision-making about your own health.

It is no longer the case that knowledge about human health is the exclusive domain of medical professionals. We don't need to rely solely on a practitioner to dispense a treatment plan and dollops of information that might simply align with their own personal and professional world view. Today we can take our health in our own hands.

Don't get me wrong; medical and other healthcare professionals are central to the operation of a successful healthcare system and, ultimately, to your health and longevity. But now, more than ever before, you can gain the knowledge relevant to your own health that puts you in the driver's seat.

The ready availability of medical knowledge is accelerating scientific progress, and it is empowering individuals to take control of their own treatment programmes. But the greatest benefit of the information age is that, by accruing more knowledge about your body and health, you will be better able to tap into an inner well of healing power. With this knowledge you can leverage the strange phenomena of quantum physics and become what is called the Quantum Observer. (More on this later.)

When it comes to cardiovascular health, nobody but you can appreciate the awesome power of the heart and its ability to overcome the forces of ill health.

A new evidence-based, holistic model is ready to be downloaded to the DNA to empower it and to promote beneficial change. A new, cardio centred model is necessary for each of us to comprehend the field of holistic heart health and medical physics of the 21st century. The accelerating pace of change in medical science and the expansion of medical physics can create a win/win situation for everybody.

Conventional western medicine has always taught that our bodies are mostly fixed in form and largely unchangeable. Apart from obvious things like weight gain and loss or changes in strength and flexibility, for the most part it has been accepted that our organs don't really change except for deterioration associated with ageing. It is only recently that scientists have discovered, for example, that our brains are "plastic" (changeable) and can, with some effort, recover from injury or illness. In this book you will see that many other parts and functions of our bodies are plastic; hearts, lungs and other organs can, with the right protocols, improve and heal.

As an autonomous individual your task is to connect with the intelligence of the heart and to comprehend its holistic relationships with your environment. Then you will be able to re-assess your health and put your intelligent heart at the centre of your life.

Holistic medicine and medical physics have identified six major components within the human body that are the building blocks of health. They function synergistically to map bodily awareness and spiritual consciousness. These major components maintain stable health, the growth of maturity and individual personal development.

1. The intelligent heart
2. The lungs, with the breathing mechanism
3. The quantum body, including its extended electromagnetic body field
4. The mind, brain and spinal cord
5. The genome through DNA and RNA
6. The acupuncture meridian system, the energy conduit of the human body

These six components build the visible and invisible functional circuits of the human body.

Recent discoveries and current research underline the true potential of the human heart. Modern cardiology emphasizes the heart's supreme position, as the leader of all the internal organs in the human body.

Aims of this Book

A fresh, 21st century look at heart health and a new perception of this smart internal organ is necessary on order to keep the heart healthy and to maintain a high level of intellectual wellness.

This program aims to incorporate the best of mainstream and holistic medical knowledge.

This book is a road map to holistic health. It aims to give you knowledge and tools to help you live a longer, healthier life. It will encourage you to choose the pathway of vibrant health and will help you recognise and deal with the most common medical condition in the world: quantum illness.

In these pages I set out the fundamentals of a new cardiology. By connecting with your own heart's intelligence you will access the healing strength of both your inner space and the wider cosmos. The information in this book and its practical strategies will help you to find the right holistic health care provider and give you the tools to achieve mastery over the health of your body and your life.

The pathways mapped in this book are created for everyone who is searching for holistic heart health and intellectual wellness, who wants an individualised approach to personal health instead of one-size-fits-all. The goal is for you to transition from quantum illness to sustainable health.

Book 1: The Intelligent Heart

The intelligence of the human heart builds multidimensional links to powerful domains of the body and mind. It connects you to your soul and to the domain of consciousness. The intelligent heart challenges the prevailing illness-oriented mind-set that is bound to the logic of mechanical cause and effect.

"The heart isn't mushy or sentimental. It's intelligent and powerful, and we believe that it holds the promise for the next level of human development and for the survival of our world."
Doc Childre and Howard Martin in
The HeartMath Solution

The heart's intelligence has many facets. Just like the brain, the heart is bristling with neurons – the cells that drive our thoughts and actions, our memory, emotions, movement and perception. In fact, the heart is endowed with more neurons than any other organ apart from the brain. And, just like the brain, the heart's localized nervous network manages a multitude of functions in addition to pumping blood. In its own way the heart is conscious, thinking and directing things within itself and beyond.

But here's another aspect of the heart's intelligence. Consider an astonishing 2000 study that argues that characteristics of the personality of a heart donor can be transferred to the heart transplant recipient. Paul Pearsall and colleagues at the University of Hawaii and University of Arizona Tucson interviewed ten heart transplant recipients and their families and, crucially, they interviewed relatives of the donors. They found that many transplant recipients exhibited changes in personality that aligned with the personalities of their donors. In some cases recipients experienced phenomena that were strongly suggestive of actual memories from the life of the donor. The authors said, "Parallels included changes in food, music, art, sexual, recreational, and career preferences, as well as specific instances of perceptions of names and sensory experiences related to the donors." The prevalence of these changes was such that they could not be explained by coincidence alone.

So, in addition to its roles in pumping blood and coordinating critical functions around the body, the heart's intelligence runs deeper: the heart knows things, it feels things, and it remembers.

1. About the Human Heart

We believe that we are well equipped for this new sci-tech world and that we are ready for the next level of advanced technological development. But our hearts need help to manage the demands of a 24/7 lifestyle and the explosion of data.

The heart is the most important organ of your body and it works hard to overcome Earth's gravity. Your body is situated in 3D space-time, the operational domain of the human mind. The mind directs life activities in 3D space-time and maps a hologram of the whole body within the brain.

The Majesty of the Human Heart

The heart's intelligence is encoded within its structure and functions. Its first beat occurs in the mother's womb about 10 days after conception. This tiny heart performs on a miraculous scale, beating with relentless perseverance and synchronization right through the trauma of birth and beyond, for a full lifetime.

Your heart performs the most extraordinary tasks in unison with the rest of your body, soul, mind and spirit. In the wider world, your heart interconnects with all those who make up your social network: your family and friends, professional colleagues and others. In fact, your heart is interconnected with every living being on this planet, and with the quantum world that underlies the fabric of the Universe.

The human heart can spontaneously dissolve blockages or resolve spasms in a coronary artery. And this can happen without external interventions like angioplasty balloon catheters. Part of the heart's intelligence involves dealing with these threats as they arise on a daily basis. To do this essential maintenance work, the heart must be supplied with sufficient oxygen, pure water and vital minerals such as Potassium and Magnesium. When these fundamentals are in place, the heart can often correct an irregular heart rate spontaneously.

Our hearts are subject to a constant cascade of stress, but they are equipped to deal with this on a business-as-usual basis, behind the scenes. And it is all done by means of four vital heart hormones that are released, as and when needed, every 24 to 48 minutes.

The majesty of the human heart manifests in a grand multilevel performance by:

- Beating 41 million times a year in a highly variable rhythm.
- Generating a powerful electromagnetic field inside and outside the body.
- Supplying our whole body with energy capable of delivering the electricity for a 100 watt bulb at peak performance.
- Producing precise, rhythmic contractions all day, every day, to pump the equivalent of 7,000 litres of blood throughout the body, supplying sufficient blood to all organs against the forces of gravity.
- Dynamically adjusting the heart's pumping function to the changing demands of the body and surrounding environment.
- Radically calibrating the amount of blood that is ejected in a each heartbeat.
- Building up to 3 kilograms and more of renewable energy every 24 hours, 7 days a week, in the cells of the heart.
- Producing stem cells for restoring and healing, in response to the ongoing regenerative demands of the heart itself and of the entire body
- Generally healing the embattled human heart.

The Heart is the Primary Organ

The heart is superior to other internal organs because of its multi-level governing functions at the electromagnetic, hormonal and genetic level. The heart is a sophisticated bio-engine operating in a strong electromagnetic field. It has an executive impact on all the cells of the human body.

The highest expression of general health, and heart health in particular, is radiance – an intense light around the body that emanates from within. It is a sparking, photo-bionic energy that arises from invisible, highly energised communication between cells.

The Human Heart is Created from a Single Cell

The human heart is the first organ to develop in the embryo. The heart begins to form in the womb in the 10th and 11th day of life, even before the brain. The precise functioning of the baby's heart is fundamental to the whole pregnancy and the embryo's development. The human heart is a whole, functional organ from the very beginning. It is interconnected with the mother and, even at this earliest stage, with the intangible territory of the inner and outer space of the person. The small heart of the developing baby shares in the mother's the electromagnetic body field, her blood and their common DNA.

The human heart is not created to be alone; it loves to be interconnected and to communicate with other intelligent human hearts. The developing baby is entangled, interconnected with other human hearts. It links especially to its parents' hearts and to the hearts of other family members. It is connected to loved ones and friends, even over great distances and different time zones. It never exists alone. It is fundamentally interrelated with all human beings.

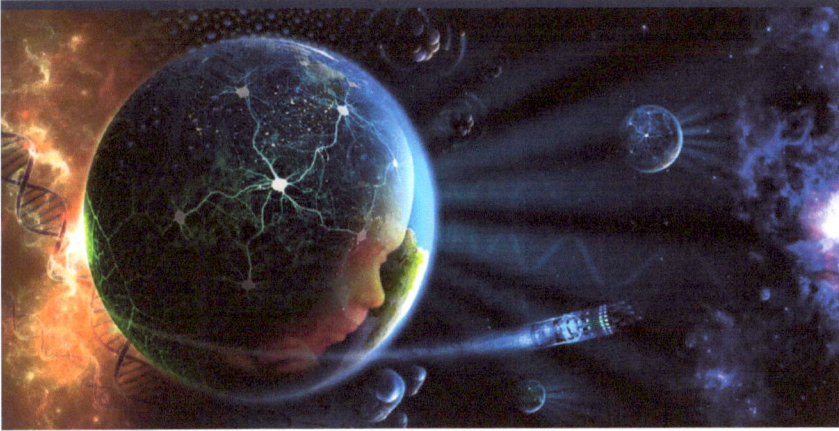

Figure 1 The image was created by US Astronaut Dr Story Musgrave MD, who has repaired the Hubble Telescope in space. Musgrave said, "It illustrates the evolution of complexity on our planet, mother Earth". It is reproduced with Dr Story permission

The Human Heart in Action

The intelligent human heart is in constant movement and communication with the body and the external environment, gathering life-giving information from inner and outer space. It translates this information and is highly responsive to the strangest, most unpredictable events. It continuously adjusts the body's blood supply by modifying the ejection fraction – the amount of blood pumped with every heartbeat. When it relaxes, the heart is filled with about 100 ml of fresh, oxygenated blood. After the ejection of the blood into aorta the remaining residual blood volume of about 45 mL stays in the left ventricle and supplies the heart itself, via the coronary artery system.

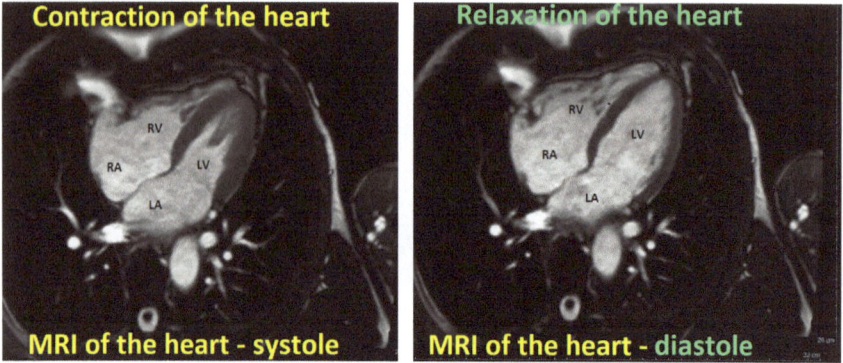

Figure 2 This MRI image shows two sequenced stages of the left chamber of the heart, in relaxation and contraction. LV is an abbreviation for the left ventricle (chamber). LA is left atrium. RV is the right ventricle and RA is the right atrium, own work

The human heart processes a vast stream of big data. It analyses this data and transforms it into useful information. The heart uses this data to constantly calibrate the ideal amount of fresh blood injected into the brain and to other vital organs, according to their actual requirements. The adjustments are based on the actual the capability of the heart itself and the capacity of the cardiovascular circulation.

The volume of blood pumped with each single heart beat has a direct effect on your physical fitness and intellectual performance. You can maximize your ejection fraction from 50 ml to 70 or even 80 ml, by practicing respiratory muscle training. This is the way that many professional athletes achieve peak performance. A slower heart rate but increased volume with every heart beat allows the body to achieve extraordinary performance. The untrained and unconditioned heart responds to every increase in emotional or bodily workload with an accelerated heart rate; but at the same time the amount of blood ejected per beat remains constant. Cardiologists now believe that this type of blood flow regulation is likely to shorten the life span.

The intelligent human heart processes electromagnetic and mechanically coded information in a far more complex and sophisticated way than previously thought. The intelligence of our heart not only maintains life but also shapes its future.

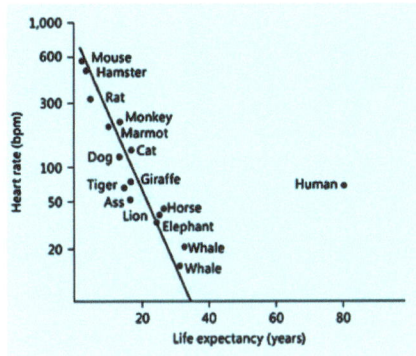

Figure 3 The diagram is shows "Heart rate, life expectancy and the cardiovascular system" of selected mammals and the humans
Courtesy: K. Boudoulas and his team from the Ohio State University

Cardiac Syndrome X in Women

It was once the case that women lived longer than men and, in particular, were less susceptible to cardiovascular disease than men. This was largely due to the protective effects of circulating hormones like oestrogens and progesterone. But over time the gap is closing. Heart attack is no longer a man's disease. In fact, cardiovascular disease is the number one killer of women now. Heart disease currently claims the lives of more than a half a million females in the USA every year. And 64% of women who die suddenly from cardiovascular disease have no previous heart symptoms. Many of these deaths can be prevented if the dysfunctional state of the heart is identified and addressed.

Cardiac syndrome X commonly affects women's health and is usually caused by the spasm of a coronary artery. CSX is associated with hormone imbalances, especially low levels of progesterone, and diminished production of heart hormones. This, in turn, is associated with repeatedly induced fight-or-flight stress responses. A lack of exercise or, conversely, too-intense physical training can also put you at higher risk of CSX.

CSX in women is also associated with a lower pain threshold, making the patient more susceptible to pain. The low pain threshold produces burning sensations and discomfort in the chest and often a real heartache. It is often incorrectly interpreted as acid reflux and heartburn but it is not related to stomach hyperacidity. It is angina pectoris. Chest discomfort is an important symptom of a temporary dysfunction caused by a spasm of the coronary artery.

Overactive adrenals and insufficient amounts of protective heart hormones can trigger an imbalance of the cardiovascular system.

Both factors can be powerful catalysts for CSX. An overactive stress cascade involves increased production of adrenaline, noradrenaline and angiotensinogen II (AT II). Angiotensinogen is one of the systemic stress hormones involved in the development of high blood pressure, causing damage to the lining of the coronary vessels. The stressful fight-or-flight response suppresses the deep abdominal breathing mechanism and causes a low level of oxygenation; which is an additional trigger of CSX.

Fight-or-Flight Response

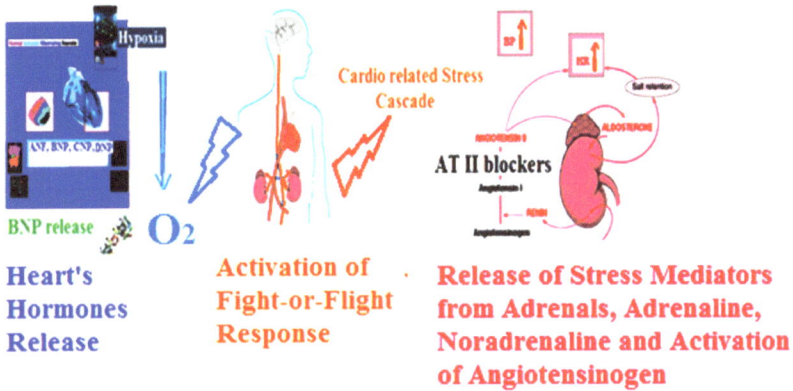

Heart's Hormones Release

Activation of Fight-or-Flight Response

Release of Stress Mediators from Adrenals, Adrenaline, Noradrenaline and Activation of Angiotensinogen

Figure 4 Interactions between the protective heart hormones, especially BNP, and the systemic fight-or-flight stress response, also involving adrenals and kidneys. BP stands for blood pressure, HR for heart rate and hypoxia means a substantial lack of oxygen

Own work

A range of agents that block AT II production are used in the treatment of CSX and other heart dysfunctions, including high blood pressure. An AT II blocker intervenes in the fight-or-flight response but it does not increase the oxygen supply.

A potential breakthrough in the treatment of CSX and the weakened heart focuses on prolonging the action of heart hormones. A new technological and pharmaceutical development published first in 2014 is a major step forward in the treatment of chronic and emerging heart weakness. This treatment aims to keep the four heart hormones biologically active for longer.

Each of the four heart hormones gives a specific protection for the cardiovascular system. These heart hormones have only a short period of bioactivity in the circulation. In fact the effective protection of heart hormones lasts 24 to 48 minutes after their release into the blood. All four heart hormones are broken down and eliminated from the circulation by the action of a chemical called neprilysin. Scientists are searching for medications that will inhibit the production of neprilysin, and thus retard the process of the elimination of the heart hormones. This is an exciting new approach that aims to support the body's own healing processes.

A new drug branded as Entresto was introduced in 2015 by Novartis, a leading 21st century pharmaceutical company. Entresto is a hybrid weapon. It has the conventional ATII blocker and has another active component, Sacubitril, which allows the heart hormones to exercise their multiple protective functions longer.

John J.V. McMurray and his team published the results of a study in *The New England Journal of Medicine* which included 8,442 patients over 27 months. The group receiving Entresto experienced 20% reduced mortality. The trial was so successful that it had to be stopped before reaching the study endpoints, for ethical reasons; the team felt they could no longer withhold this life-saving treatment from the control cohort in the trial.

A landmark 2015 study, called PARADIGM-HF was the largest clinical trial ever conducted in the weakness of the heart. The study results have shown 20% reduction of mortality in the trial group compared with the control group. The improvement of life span was mainly attributed to reduction of abnormal heart rhythms, ventricular arrhythmias and sudden cardiac death (SCD).

Recycling Stress Hormones using the Intelligence of the Heart

We each have a gene called COMT which performs miracles when we're under physical or emotional stress. COMT governs a process whereby the heart's cells neutralise the negative effects of stress hormones. The letter O in the enzyme COMT stands for oxygen, because oxygen accelerates the recycling process. And this explains the connection between the intensity of our breathing and the effects of the stress response in our body.

The object in red, above, is a molecule of the stress hormone Adrenaline in its active form. The green molecule is an inactivated hormone ready to be re-used.

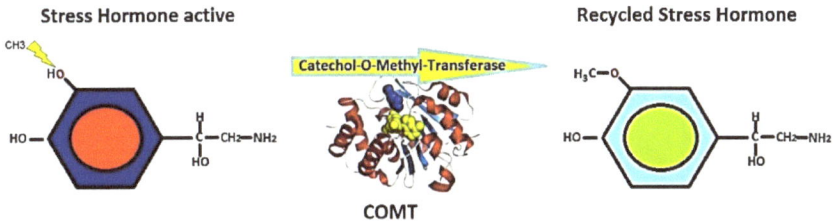

Recycling of Stress Hormones in the Blood Circulation

Figure 5 Recycling of stress hormones
own work

Using this recycling process, the heart neutralizes the negative effects of stress mediators, converting them into an efficient fuel to be converted into cellular energy.

7TM Receptors

Intense communication within the body and with the direct environment happens via specific cellular structures known as receptors. The heart is connected to the interior of the body and to the external environment via special 7TM receptors. These receptors act like a cellular smart phone, receiving and sending signals and messages about external electromagnetic, thermic and mechanical influences, about pulsating waves, blood pressure, mechanical vibrations. All these factors are triggers and cause a release of the heart hormones produced in the chambers and released in the circulation.

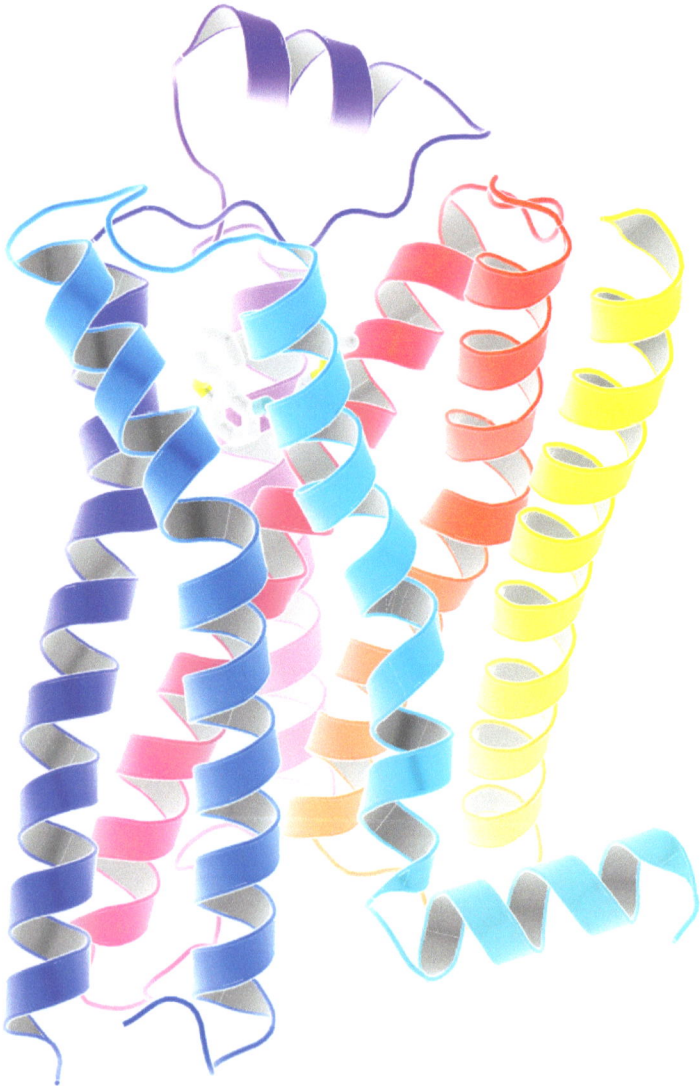

Figure 6 Displays one of the 7TM receptors existing at cell
surface that detects molecules and electromagnetic
impulses outside the cell and activate cellular responses
Image: Wikipedia Commons, by Opabinia regalis

The 7 blades of the 7TM receptor cross the cell membrane exist in
all the cells of the heart and in all other compartments of the human

body. The 7TM receptors contain two molecules of cholesterol, colored yellow, which form a micro crystal resonating with incoming and outgoing impulses and frequencies. The 7 TM receptors build an interface between the visible and invisible world. Every cell has in fact hundred thousand or more of these small antennas receiving all kind of impulses. The functions of the 7 TM receptors and light based visual perception via receptors in the eyes allow spatial orientation and the realization of the sky and space above.

Intense communication within the body and with the direct environment happens via specific cellular structures known as receptors. These cell receptors act like a cellular smart phone, receiving and sending signals and messages about external electromagnetic, thermic and mechanical influences, about pulsating waves, blood pressure, mechanical vibrations. All these factors are triggers and cause a release of heart hormones produced in the chambers and released into our blood circulation. The heart cells build mechanical, electrical and electromagnetic energy.

The 7 blades of the 7TM receptor cross the cell membrane exist in all the cells of the heart and in all other compartments of the human body. The 7TM receptors contain two molecules of cholesterol which form a micro crystal resonating with incoming and outgoing impulses and frequencies. The 7TM receptors build an interface between the visible and invisible world.

2. The Ten Levels of the Heart's Intelligence

...because you are sons, God has sent out the Spirit of his Son into our hearts, saying, Abba, Father. (Galatians 4:6)

The human heart modulates all surrounding and interfering frequencies into one understandable language of human life. It discerns the intelligent direction towards life with all its expressions. Every mechanical heartbeat initiates the heartbeat-evoked electrical potentials in the brain.

The heart knows what is right. It distinguishes between the healthy and the unhealthy tendencies in our bodies and our environment.

There are 10 levels of intelligence within the human heart that govern and fine tune its communication with other internal organs. This has a direct impact on an individual's level of harmony and wellbeing.

1. Mechanical Precision
2. Acoustic Messaging
3. Electromagnetic Function
4. Neuronal Intelligence
5. Genomic Intelligence (DNA)
6. Hormonal Dominance
7. Heart's Regenerative Power
8. Metabolic Independence
9. The Quantum Connection to the Fabric of the Universe
10. Emotional Intelligence

Mechanical precision

The heart is a phenomenal machine, coordinating blood supply throughout the entire body. It has an array of mechanical sensors, detecting impulses related to blood circulation and its smooth flow. The sensors, called receptors, are mostly located in the blood vessels and in the heart's internal walls. They instantly detect turbulence or abnormal changes inside our four heart cavities. They monitor oxygen saturation, water and minerals in the blood and blood pressure levels.

Other receptors calibrate the volume and temperature of circulating blood according to the requirements of the body. They adjust the body's pH level and correct mineral imbalances. When the receptors sense something abnormal, they release some or all of the heart's 4 hormones to prevent negative impacts. (These four heart hormones will be discussed in more detail later.)

The human heart strives after perfection at all times. It can rebalance the turbulent vortex flow produced by a temporarily rigid heart wall. It can prevent premature ventricular beats disturbing and disrupting smooth blood flow. The mechanical functions of the intelligent heart are reflected in a harmonious, smooth rhythm and in gentle pulse and pressure waves propagated all over the body. The quality of the pulse wave can be recognized by a careful examination known as pulse diagnostics.

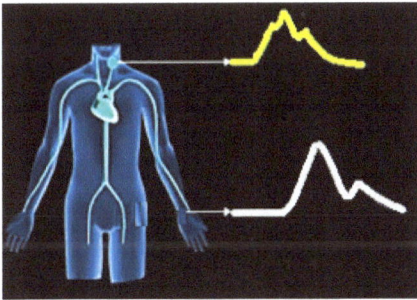

Figure 7 An example of the mechanical wave created through the heart and registered as pulse waves at the hand from the radial artery and at the neck from the carotid artery
own work

In modern medicine, pulse diagnostics involves the fingertip palpation of an artery at the wrist known as the radial artery, to detect and assess the profile of the pulse waves produced by the beating heart. The doctor will measure the heart rate and check for abnormalities in rhythm. This pulse examination may indicate any heart problems such as irregular heartbeat or palpitations. A swelling of the blood vessel can be a sign of high blood pressure.

Our regular heartbeat is generated without break for an average life span of about 80 years[. It is quite interesting that the mechanical pulse and pressure waves are the origin of the specific brain activations. The heart's mechanical waves are converted in the brain into electromagnetic activity known as the heartbeat evoked potentials.

A 2007 paper by Marcus A. Gray and Peter Taggart describes this amazing transformation.

Having been evoked in brain, these electrical potentials then travel to the spine and through the nervous system, reaching the entire body as part of the coordinated heart/brain network. It is harmonious cooperation and which evokes a dynamic response from the activated cells. The cells receive intense down-streaming informational traffic which activates the cells' 7TM receptors, resulting in activation of the DNA. In turn the DNA genetic code has to be copied and the message has to be sent to the cells. It has a helper, the news bringer, known as messenger RNA, or mRNA. These little messengers stimulate the production of hormones related to our feelings and emotions.

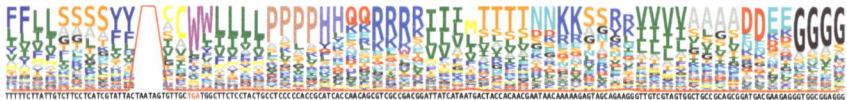

Figure 8 The Genetic code

Wikipedia Commons by Bas E. Dutilh, Rasa Jurgelenaite, Radek Szklarczyk, Sacha A.F.T. van Hijum, Harry R. Harhangi, Markus Schmid, Bart de Wild, Kees-Jan Françoijs, Hendrik G. Stunnenberg, Marc Strous, Mike S.M. Jetten, Huub J.M. Op den Camp and Martijn A. Huynen

All of this amounts to a living and pulsating information cascade, starting with every heartbeat. At the same time, the inscription of these pathways is the ultimate legacy for the offspring we co-create as the next generation.

A good illustration of the role of the genetic code is presented in the illustration above.

Genetic DNA information is stored as a sequence of letters originating from four bases. The letters represent the bases: Adenine (A), Thymine (T), Guanine (G) and Cytosine (C).

In the DNA strain the letter A (Adenine) always pairs with T (Thymine), and the C letter (Cytosine) with G, standing for Guanine. In the mRNA, the letter T (Thymine} is replaced by Uracil (U).

Acoustic Messaging

Sounds are everywhere in our environment. The dominant acoustic frequencies in the modern life come with an intense power and influence the whole body. It is usually easy to recognize them and to know their origin or to decode the source of the sometimes disturbing sounds. We are used to these sounds. However it's not so easy to be aware of the sounds coming from inside of the body. The loudest bodily sound is the breath, the sound of the lungs. The specific tone of the heartbeat is very gentle. But sometimes, in cases of anxiety or exertion, the heart can pound.

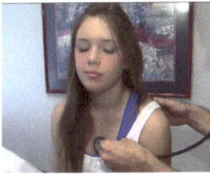

Figure 9 A general practitioner uses a stethoscope to listen to your heartbeat and the gentle sound of breathing
Wikipedia Commons, author Alith3204

The process of listening to the internal sounds of the body, "auscultation", is one of the basic methods of assessing the heart. Your doctor can hear the valves opening and closing, and the acoustic phenomena of blood moving through blood vessels.

The sounds of the heart were first scientifically described by Sir Thomas Lewis, an English cardiologist and a scientist, in 1920. In the same year he published the book: *The Mechanism and Graphic Registration of the Heart Beat.*

An electronic stethoscope, which is a 21st century tool of auscultation, provides excellent acoustic amplification of the heart's sounds, which can also be made audible to the patient.

A healthy heart produces two sounds. The first heart sound is created by contraction of the heart and the ejection of the blood .The second sound is caused by the relaxation of the heart and the movement of the blood filling it. The heart's sounds can also be displayed as a diagram.The sounds made by the beating heart convey valuable information about the cardiovascular system. This finding is set out in a 2012 paper called "Discovery of multiple level heart-sound morphological variability resulting from changes in physiological states."

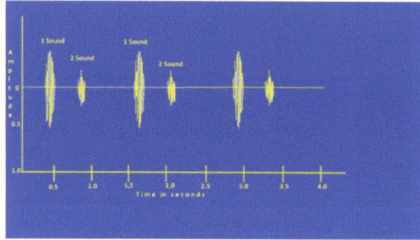

Figure 10 Two sounds of the heart
registered with microphone know as
phonocardiogram
Own work

This fascinating research brings evidence that even stem-cell production may be responding to acoustic low frequency signals produced by the heart and the vibrations of the Earth. These specific sounds affect hormone production, regeneration of tissues and the breathing mechanism, as well as the functioning of the cardiovascular system. The heart's sounds reach all cells and their DNA, initiating a stream of life-supporting impulses. It is very similar to the heart's mechanical actions reaching the brain.

Electromagnetic Function

Like everything, the human body is built from vibrating and continuously charging atoms and subatomic particles. This electromagnetic reality is grade school physics, but sometimes the awareness of the electromagnetic nature of the human body is not sufficiently taken account of when considering human health. The electrically charged nature of the particles that make up our bodies combine to create an invisible but powerful electromagnetic field that surrounds us. This field acts as a protective shield. The atoms and subatomic-particles that make up your body vibrate at a specific frequency, which is the unique signature of your "quantum body".

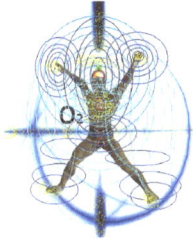

Figure 11 An artist's vision of the electromagnetic field of the human body
Own work

The constant spin of hydrogen protons is charging the field and creating electricity, the guided flow of the electrons through human body. This electrical current generated by the heart can be registered as can be electrocardiogram, in abbreviation ECG. The electrocardiogram has a QRS complex reflecting the heart's excitation and contraction and the T wave happening during the relaxation phase.

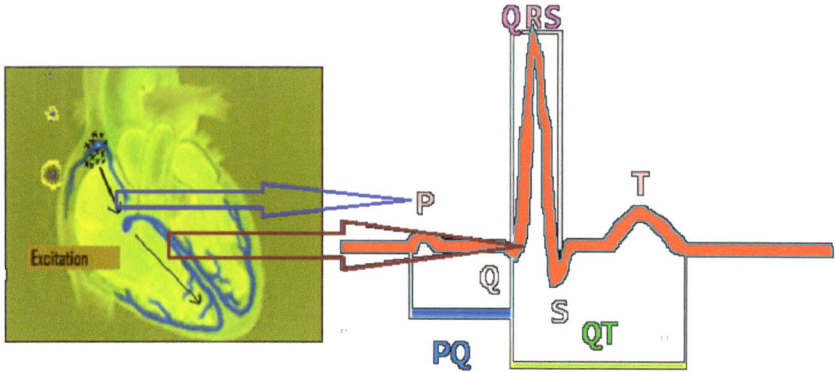

Figure 12 Electrocardiogram with its major waves P, QRS and T and their origins in the heart
Own work

Pioneering research by the HeartMath Institute of Research Centre in California, USA confirmed the existence of the morphogenetic body field. This electromagnetic field is an invisible extension of the human body and has a wireless component to it. It constitutes an informational, energetic body field based on the electromagnetic functions of the light and bio-photons spiralling from and towards the human body. Bio-photons, the smallest quanta of light, are emitted from every living system. They can be detected as a subtle but very specific biological electromagnetic radiation. The bio-photons forming the body field and electromagnetic radiation are the signs of the activity of your heart, your DNA, and your brain's activation.

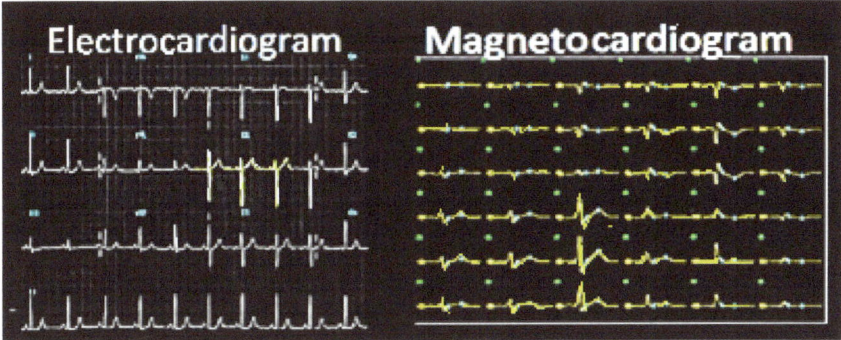

**Figure 13 Electrocardiogram (ECG) on the left side of the
picture, and the magnetocardiogram MCG the right**
Own work

The electromagnetic activity of the heart can be read for diagnostic purposes as a continuous record of repeated electrical vectors known as electrocardiogram (ECG) on the left side of the picture, or as a magnetocardiogram MCG the right side of the picture. Both look similar and have similar time characteristics during registration.

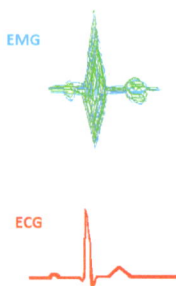

Figure 14 One full electrical cycle of a heartbeat. The electronic drawing of a modern registration of both an electrocardiogram ECG (bottom of the picture) and magnetocardiogram MCG (in the upper part)
Own work

The heart is a major contributor to our magnetic body field. It is a very sophisticated, complex system which is able to transform big data into intelligent life giving, information. The heart's electromagnetic power recharges the body field in an on-going process throughout our lives.

Each of us is involved in a virtual world and we need to counteract the influence of many artificial business models, the new societal sequencing of the media, and the difficult complex of family related matters. The complexity of these forces is growing exponentially, and their impact increasingly affects the electromagnetic field of the heart.

Neuronal Level of Intelligence

The heart and brain are the two most powerful organs working usually in precise harmony. They create coherence and determine intellectual wellness/wellbeing. The perfect communication of the heart/brain can elevate the natural mind to its highest potential.

The HeartMath Institute in California, USA performed a series of experiments on coherent heart/brain interactions, showing that the human heart contains specific neuronal tissue known "a brain in the heart". In one study the heart and brain of a subject were wired for measurement. Devices registered both the heart's and the brain's electromagnetic response. The subject sat in front of a screen. Random selected images were displayed without any sequence. The pictures ranged from very pleasant to the most terrifying situations. Amazingly, the heart responded first. What most astonished the researchers was the fact that the heart reacted to the images even before they appeared on the screen.

This experiment confirmed the electromagnetic intelligence of the heart. It was capable of responding to the images independent of and prior to the brain. Sometimes, the heart allows a person to anticipate a glimpse of the future event in a way that is not possible for the five senses and brain's perception. In contrast, when these two pivotal organs are not properly synchronised, the result is dysfunctional concentration, poor memory and a mental discomfort because of the blood supply restrictions to the brain.

Insufficient blood supply to the brain can cause a syndrome known as a "selfish brain". This is an effort of the restricted brain to gain more energy in an emergency. The brain can use all available neuronal regulations and the hormonal influence of the pituitary gland to direct blood supply and streams of energy to itself. The selfish action of the brain poses risks, and can be life threatening if the intelligent heart does not intervene.

A perfectly functioning heart is the ultimate safeguard of your general health. The intelligent heart exercises its neuronal superiority in two ways: it uses its own, fully independent nervous system, and can release specific hormones to calibrate the blood supply to the brain. Only a healthy heart and a properly functioning cardiovascular system can equip the human body to face the unpredictable challenges of modern life.

Genomic Intelligence (DNA)

The heart's genomic wisdom can secure long lasting endurance and optimal functioning. This genomic capability can sustain the heartbeat for the life span of 100, sometimes up to 120, years.

An analysis of the genes coding the heart in in harmony with the body's genome shows more than 60% of all human genes for the production of proteins are strongly expressed in the heart itself. Importantly, 248 genes which control protein production are expressed in the heart significantly more than in other internal organs.

There are also 120 special genes sharing information between the heart and other internal organs, including especially the brain. The heart governs a big and complex genetic network.

Of the three billion letters that make up the entire human genome, only 15 million (1/60,000 of the full genome) are specific to humans. This is a tiny fraction. These human-specific genetic regions are known as the human accelerated regions (HARs). They make our own genome strikingly different from all other animals.

Professor Katherine Pollard from the University of California in San Francisco, USA was the first scientist to discover and describe the human accelerated regions (HARs) in 2006.

Oxygen

Oxygen is essential for protein production, including in the heart and brain. The brain can hardly survive more than 3 to 5 minutes without oxygen. It is obvious that appropriate genetic coding for optimal breathing and a freshly oxygenated blood supply is a matter of the highest priority.

Humans are highly dependent on sufficient oxygenation of the body. Our bodies are able to adjust our metabolism according to level of available oxygen. Your body has two kinds of metabolism, **foetal metabolism** and **adult metabolism**. Foetal metabolism operates ideally in an oxygen-poor environment, and is operational during embryonic development in the womb. Foetal metabolism is 80% sugar based and only 20% based on fat (fatty acids). Fat produces a limited amount of energy for the cells, which is sufficient to survive in the womb, Adult metabolism took over after you were born, and is tuned for survival in an oxygen-rich environment. Unlike foetal metabolism, adult metabolism is 80% fat based and 17 times more efficient than the foetal metabolism in producing energy. The adult metabolism is only found in humans.

PPARγ and HARs

The heart has a genetic switcher between foetal metabolism, and adult metabolism. The switcher between these two kinds of metabolism is the PPARγ gene, the peroxisome proliferator-activated receptor.

The author published a study about the prevalence of the active form of this gene PPARγ, which is abundantly present in the human accelerated region (HAR) gene of the heart. The results suggested this genetic switcher between foetal and adult metabolism it is weakened in its functionality because of insufficient oxygenation.

Professor Pollard's colleagues also found that the HARs evolved four times faster than other genetic regions. These specific changes in the human gene lineage represent a unique step in human development. They suggest that our hearts are well equipped for the challenges of our multitasking 21st century lifestyle.

Another group of scientists led by Capra found that HARs are developmental enhancers. The Capra group found in 2014 that 251 of the 773 HARs enhancers are active in brain development, 194 are active in limb development and 39 are active in heart development. This acceleration of enhancers for the brain and limbs is caused by the need to adapt to our rapidly changing environment, with many factors influencing the brain/mind functionality and the functions of the hands. While the majority of HAR enhancers are active in only one of the organs, 50 have been assigned to two organs/tissues. Interestingly, the team identified only one multifunctional gene enhancer. It originates in the heart and is very active across three locations: heart, brain and limbs.

The relative low number of enhancers for the heart reflects the fact the heart's developmental process is older than the brain's. The heart is the first organ formed in embryonic development in the uterus. It is already a mature organ at the very early stages of the human life.

High data traffic in the DNA of the heart and brain can cause informational overload. A rapid DNA dysfunction can be triggered through low oxygenation and overactive stress responses. If these two triggers continue too long, the result may be the development of neuro-degenerative disorders like Parkinson's or Alzheimer's disease.

The brain is genetically less equipped than the heart in survival situations. The heart can renew and protect itself even in extremely unfavourable conditions including poor blood and oxygen supply.

The Hibernating Heart

The intelligent heart has a special set of genes to deal with an oxygen crisis like Broken Heart Syndrome. The lack of oxygen due to a blockage or a spasm of the coronary artery is a strong signal for the heart to protect itself through hibernation (hibernating myocardium), reducing the blood supply to the affected area of the heart to the survival level. At the same time the heart's DNA increases the gene expression of the hypoxia induced factor (HIF). The Hypoxia gene that is activated in a low oxygenation emergency helps to protect and sustain hibernating myocardium as long as possible until the obstruction of the coronary artery is resolved. HIF substantially mitigates the damage caused by low oxygenation. Hibernation can continue for a short or long time. For this reason the heart has a perfect time measure mechanism. - a genetic clock supporting the heart in its ability to overcome emergencies caused through low oxygenation. In genetic terms the supressing negative influence of a special gene known as the "circadian locomotors outcome cycles kaput" (CLOCK) will be put on hold and all emergency energy resources are open to bypass the obstruction. The CLOCK gene is designed for extremely distressing situations and is designed to preserve energy resources. It down-regulates energy production through the whole body, and prepares the heart for with the more critical situations to come.

When a risk factor triggers a negative energy loop it initiates in a person the feeling of being powerless and lacking of energy. Sometimes the acceleration of a stressful situation pushes the heart to the very edge. The stored energy in the body will allow an individual to perform extraordinary feats. The affected person can sometimes go far beyond her/his physical and mental capacity. Suddenly a person at the frontier between life and death is able to overcome extraordinary, life threatening circumstances.

After this extraordinary performance the heart's CLOCK gene usually returns to normal operation. The return of the positive energy feedback loop restores calm and lets the individual forget the life threatening storm.

Hormonal Dominance

The heart's hormones have effects throughout the body and sustain its integrity in normal and stressful conditions. These four hormones preserve, protect and support multiple bodily functions. Their functionality goes far beyond their impact on metabolism, energy production. They affect the stress response, fat metabolism, blood acidity/alkalinity, the equilibrium of tissue oxygenation and the water/minerals balance.

The intelligent heart produces four major independent hormones: the atrial natriuretic peptide type A, brain natriuretic peptide type B, the type C, which was first discovered in salmon and the type D, which is similar to a hormone found in a snake known as the green mamba, They make up the natriuretic peptide family.

The heart's hormones accelerate energy production of adenosine tri-phosphate (ATP) to fuel cellular breathing. Inhaled oxygen converts adenosine di-phosphate (ADP) (a lower level energy carrier) into the high energy ATP, available for all the cells of the human body.

In emergency situations the intelligent heart can produce two further hormones, cardiomyosin and serum response factor, which reduce blood supply to the brain when it demands too much energy. This occurs when the imbalanced situation between heart/brain continues for too long. These two emergency hormones will be released when the brain becomes selfish and demands more and more energy at the cost of the heart, and at the cost of the other internal organs.

The elevated levels of both of these hormones are found in Alzheimer's disease and dementia and they are associated with brain degeneration.

The Heart's Regenerative Power

Our hearts are designed to work continuously for over 80 years. They require continuous and powerful regeneration. Every heart produces adult omnipotent stem cells. This astonishing fact was discovered in 2010 at Harvard University. Adult omnipotent stem cells regenerate and restore damaged heart tissue as part of the heart's normal, lifelong operation, and without us even noticing.

A growing body of evidence suggests that all internal organs possess similar regenerative potential. This discovery was a revolutionary step in regenerative medicine and the 2012 Nobel Prize was awarded to John B. Gurdon and Dr Shinya Yamanaka for their research showing that mature cells can be reprogrammed to become omnipotent adult stem cells for all internal organs of the human body. The ability to produce adult omnipotent stem cells by the liver, kidney, spleen and other internal organs is one of the key factors in the body's capacity for lifelong renewal. This breakthrough research confirmed that even so called slow speed regenerative organs such as the heart (it needs in average 20 years for the complete renewal) and brain (it needs about 40 years for exchange of all nerve cells) can heal and regenerate. The human heart can regenerate even its own sensors, the 7TM cell receptors, according to the needs of cells.

The Quantum Connection to the Fabric of the Universe

The quantum connection of the heart refers to its relationship with the invisible world of subatomic particles and the unlimited potentiality waves which together constitute the fabric of the Universe. Throughout history the heart was considered a place of love, compassion, intuition and wisdom. The heart has been seen as a gateway to consciousness, truth and a spiritual connection with the unseen world. However, life in 3D space-time is mostly experienced with the five general senses.

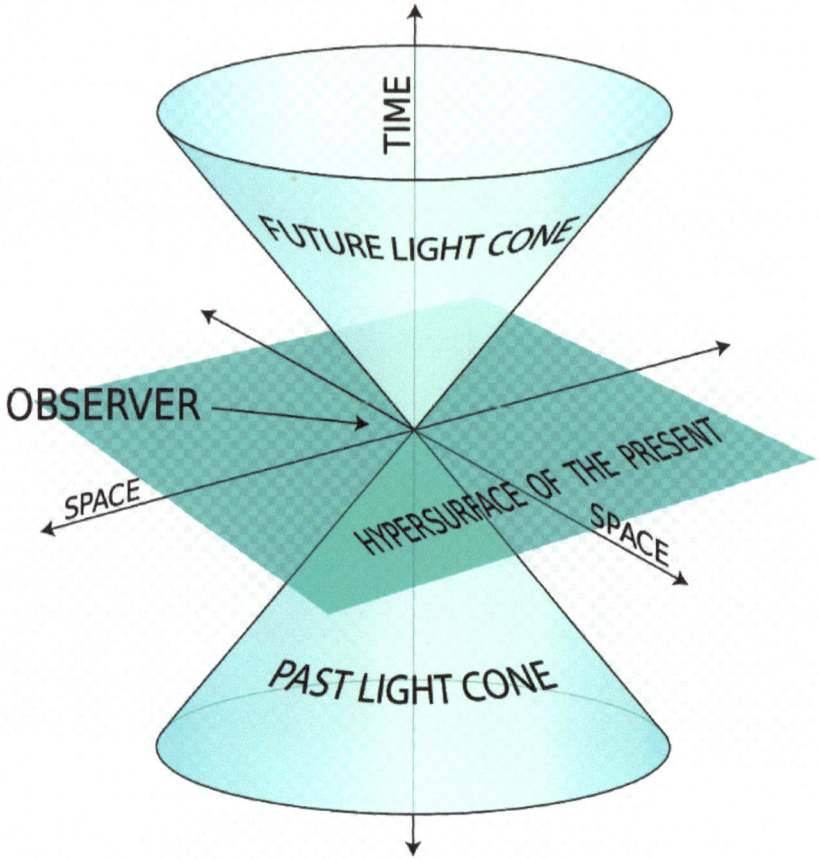

Figure 15 Two-dimensional space depicted in
three-dimensional space-time. The past and future light
cones are absolute, the "present" is a relative concept
different for observers in relative motion
Wiki Commons by K. Aainsqatsi

The heart is a sensitive organ, a knowledgeable instrument and a great tool to explore and map the invisible worlds beyond visible reality.

The heart is the biggest contributor to the body's magnetic field and the most precise mediator of these invisible connections. The body's field is an interface between the individual and the quantum environment. The heart communicates with probability waves. It is known in medical physics as the quantum probability approach.

This invisible world of small particles, super symmetry and probability waves can be explored by way of the heart and spirit. Both map invisible quantum reality and build a grid for holistic consciousness.

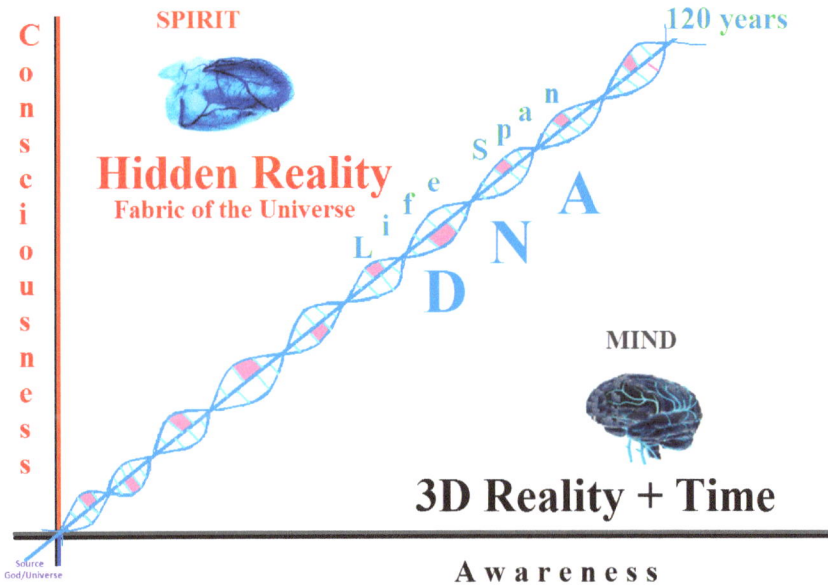

Figure 16 The human body is holistically designed for exploring invisible electromagnetic reality, the functions of the spirit by the heart and the functioning of the awareness in the 3 D reality by the brain/mind. The duration of the individual life span displayed as the DNA line relates to the balance between operational, spiritual activity in the hidden reality of the fabric of the Universe and the actions in the solid 3D reality

Own work

The Superior Mind

The mind and the brain cooperate with the heart. Together they build special functions known as the superior mind.

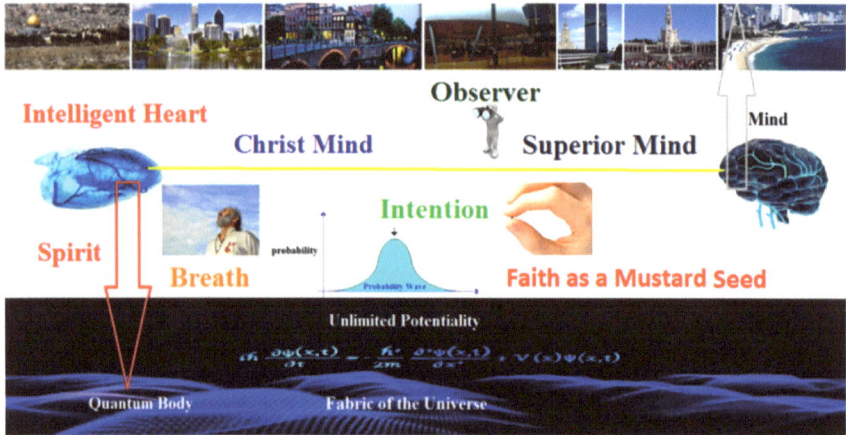

17. The spirit explores the spiritual, invisible and hidden electromagnetic dimension, and builds the grid for the operations of consciousness. The strongest power is attributed to the intention

Own work

The superior mind knows 3D space-time; it comprehends touchable and invisible realities. It is the perfect mind, grounded in the heart's intelligence and its connections to the fabric of the Universe. The superior mind knows what is right and what is not good to do in 3D space-time. One's progress in life depends on the right balance between 3D space-time and the fabric of the Universe. And that is the domain of the heart and the spirit, as shown in the timeline of the DNA displayed above.

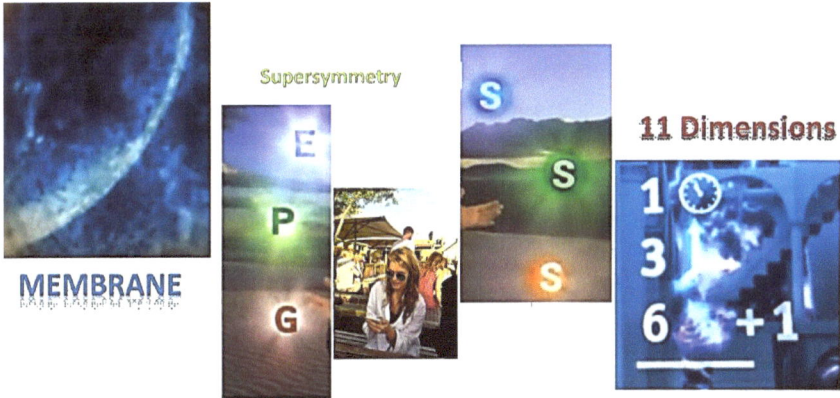

Figure 18 The supersymetry in the universe and in nature empowers our fundamental understanding of the cosmos, from the universality of gravity to the unification of the forces of nature at higher energy levels. The letter E stands for electron, P for proton. G for gravity and the related three s letters are symbolically the predicted super symmetry particles
Own work with four extracts of the images from the documentary film The Elegant Universe: Welcome to the 11th Dimension by Dr Brian Greene

The human electromagnetic body field constitutes a shield against the powerful geo-influences and gravity of our planet. It can cooperate with the fabric of the Universe and with the invisible worlds of super-strings, membranes in space, and the super symmetry.

Emotional Intelligence

Emotional intelligence according to Doug Ramsay's definition: :Emotional intelligence EI can be defined as one's ability to observe, detect, and categorize one's own emotions as well as those of others, while using this information to inform one's decisions, thinking, and behaviour." is a capacity which can be developed by the heart and its intelligence. By using our innate EI, it is possible to recognize our own systemic response to the emotions arising from the holistic systems of the body, and to interpret other people's emotions. Emotional intelligence allows you to differentiate between related feelings and to decode them. The feelings are the feedback. This is a helpful message from the Universe. If we are good in the vast plane of our thoughts, the Universe confirms it and helps us to create good feelings. EI is the underlying driver of human communication and our communication with the Universe. The heart uses emotional intelligence to navigate the social and geopolitical environment. The term emotional intelligence first appeared in a 1964 paper by Michael Beldoch, its popularity rose after the publication of the book in the 1995 by Daniel Goleman, a psychologist and a science journalist of the New York Times. EI is placed between consciousness and awareness and can operate in both 3D space-time and in the 5th electromagnetic invisible dimension.

Emotions can trigger violent responses found in inter-generational junk DNA. Love seems to be the highest expression of our emotional intelligence. Love can create an unrestricted access to the 5th electromagnetic dimension and the fabric of the Universe.

The Intelligent Heart's Multi Level Communication

The heart is in constant movement and hyper busy, executing smart communication with our internal organs, tissues and the external environment. The 7TM receptor is a multipurpose sensor/receptor acting as a receiver for all kinds of wave frequencies. These frequencies originate from outside the body – like sounds, light or electromagnetic waves – and they carry specific information which can be decoded by the 7TM receptor.

Analogue, rhythmic cycles reflect mechanical, biochemical, thermic and electromagnetic functions in the body. They can be converted to electrical signals and recorded like waves, as in the electrocardiogram (ECG).

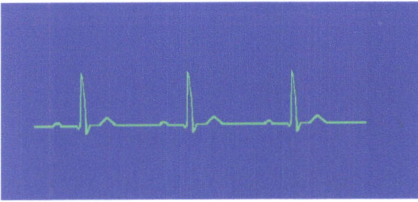

Figure 19 Analogue, rhythmic cycles such as the electrocardiogram ECG are fundamental for dynamic interactions in the human body
Own work

Human body body generates massive amounts of data – big biological data – which expresses information about its state. The body's temperature, the speed of blood flow, blood pressure, a laminar or turbulent blood flow, movements of the fluid in the spine and brain, the sound of the heart beat and the human voice all have an analogue nature. But they can be observed, recorded and quantified, and expressed as useful data. A good example of a record of analogue information is a 24-hour measurement showing highs and lows of the blood pressure.

Note that the recorded blood pressure always remains within a given range; it never reaches zero. If it ever did, the patient would be dead.

In contrast, the digital flow of information is characterized by computer coding of all signals with "0" and "1". The most distinctive difference between digital and analogue data is that the digital signal is not continuous. There is a break, a pause, in-between the digital items.

If we apply the digital flow of information to the biological system of the body it could express both: 1 for life and 0 for death. All kinds of electronic equipment can interpret these digital impulses "1" or "0". These two digits represent two opposite states and they are radically different from each other. Digital signals are used for computing and for artificial intelligence (AI).

Your intelligent heart communicates in an analogue, wave-based continuous way. It connects humans to the world of sounds and electromagnetic fields. It also creates the feelings of love and empathy, and connects the human body to the probability waves of the fabric of the Universe. It communicates with other internal organs without break and also exchanges information with other hearts. The intelligent heart communicates 24/7 with our DNA, brain and other internal organs continuously with varying intensity and never makes a stop, an interruption.

The brain uses different carriers of information: electromagnetic waves, neuronal electricity, hormones, bio-photons, the smallest particles of light, bio-chemicals, small molecules such as nitric oxide (NO), or oxygen (O2), pulse propagation waves and blood pressure. The brain communicates life.

The cyclic nature of our breath supports the dynamic world of the beating heart. Our rhythmic breath, the pulsation of life, is a vivid connection to the external world and our environment. If the breath loses its strength and does not deliver enough oxygen to the heart, the intelligent heart will protect itself. It restricts the blood supply to the brain and enters a protective state of hibernation. Otherwise the heart cells would die.

The Intelligent Heart Is Linked to Memory

Memory is one of the most sophisticated functions of humans, creating a big part of your personality. A study conducted and published in 2000 by Pearsall P. at al. made it evident that our heart is linked to memory. The study delivered astonishing evidence that a part of a donor's personality can be present in the memory and awareness of heart transplant recipients.

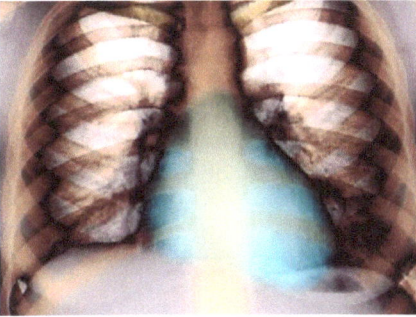

Figure 20 The result of chronic heart failure is an enlarged heart.as seen in this chest x-ray. Enlargement can also be detected by means of an ultrasound or MRI scan
Own work

The study revolutionized the way we perceive the heart and its intelligence. Recipients of transplanted hearts remembered specific life circumstances of the donors; despite never having had any contact with them. This was modern science's acknowledgment of the heart as an extremely sensitive organ, inheriting our memories.A weak heart is one of the most important contributors to poor memory. A Dutch study performed by Mosterd at al. on 5,540 participants with weak hearts showed memory deficits of almost 40%. A weak heart cannot supply the brain with sufficient blood and oxygen.

A 2014 study made by Leto L. at al. examining patients with weak or enlarged hearts showed that heart failure is associated with a 67% increased risk of cognitive impairment.

Memory problems relate to a weak heart and this is an extremely important factor in planning medical care.

According to another 2008 study performed by Sauvé M.J. at al. showed that in more than half of patients with heart weakness have problems with memory and with the other aspects of intellectual functioning.

3. The Heart's Hormones

The breakthrough discovery that opened the way to research into the heart's intelligence was the 1980 identification of a heart hormone. Researchers realised that the heart generates its own hormones, and this triggered a paradigm change. This discovery overturned the traditional mechanical perception of the heart. It shifted the heart from the position of a mechanical pump to an intelligent organ, sensing and reacting intelligently to different conditions within and outside the body.

The heart generates four hormones, each of which is a multilevel, multitasking messenger, working to mitigate proliferating stress cascades. These four compounds help to maintain a smooth and harmonious heart rhythm. They regulate blood supply to all our organs and tissues, and cooperate with our genes. It's these bio-chemical and genetic interactions that govern the heart's responses to changes in the circadian day/night cycle.

If your heart hormones are in short supply, this can have a serious impact on cardiovascular health.

Your heart releases its hormones every 24 or 48 minutes, no matter if you are healthy or ill, busy or resting. Among their multitude of functions, your heart hormones:

- Support the detoxification process and regulate the generation of Adenosine triphosphate ATP which is a primary driver of energy for all the cells in your body. By regulating the levels of ATP, the heart's hormones facilitate cellular detoxification – enabling the removal of "stagnant water" from the cells.
- Manage blood viscosity (keeping the blood thin and fluid), ensuring sufficient blood flow to every internal organ.
- Help to keep internal conditions stable and in balance (homeostasis), including the body's pH (acid / alkaline balance).
- Protect the entire cardiovascular system and can prevent mini strokes and heart attacks.
- Combat the bio-chemical actions mediating the fight-or-flight stress response
- Can stimulate the recycling process of stress hormones, adrenaline or noradrenaline.

All four of the heart's hormones have multiple links to other hormones such as thyroxin from the thyroid gland and sex hormones such as oestrogen or progesterone.

The production and release of heart hormones are oxygen-dependent processes. Once they are released, these heart hormones only remain active in the circulation for between 24 to 48 minutes. But in the presence of abundant oxygen the heart hormones are active and effective for much longer.

Therefore, it makes good sense to consider ways to deliver maximum oxygen to your system to keep the heart hormones active for longer. Even a small increase in available energy can exponentially accelerate life-sustaining bio-chemical transformations within our cells.

The most effective method for delivering increased oxygen – and hence increased energy to the cells – is the use of diaphragmatic breathing (of which, more later).

Here is a short discussion of the roles of each of the four key heart hormones.

Heart's Hormone Type A: ANP

In 1980 Dr Adolfo J. de Bold, an Argentinean-Canadian Cardiologist discovered atrial natriuretic peptide (ANP), a hormone secreted by cells of the inner lining of the heart. This discovery opened a new era of medical research.

The discovery of the ANP type A was a game changer in the fight against cardiovascular stress. ANP is released in the left atrium of the heart in any situation where the heart muscle is not performing correctly. The release of ANP is an immediate response to any stress factor that lowers the oxygenation of the heart tissue or increases blood pressure. Increased blood pressure exerts a mechanical impact on the walls of the atrium (left upper pre-chamber) due to the initial weakness of the heart muscle. This triggers the release of ANP which in turn prompts the kidneys to eliminate waste from overloaded blood, and brings the enlarged atria back to normal state.

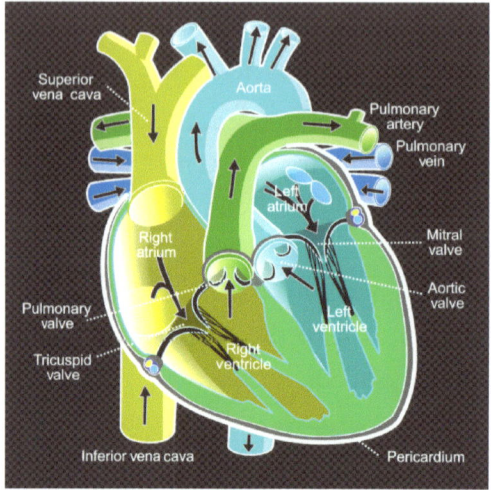

Figure 21 The anatomy of the heart showing the left atrium, where the production of adult omnipotent stem cells take place.
Wikipedia Commons by Wapcaplet

By increasing the output of ANP, the heart counteracts the enlargement of the atria and mechanical overstretching of the atrial walls.

This unhealthy force acting on the atria can cause premature heart beats or even dangerous rapid heart rate known as atrial fibrillation. A weaker heart can also reduce the blood supply to the brain.

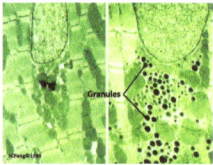

Figure 22 Atrial Natriuretic Peptide ANP granules.
Wikipedia Commons from the personal laboratory pictures of Dr Pang

This negative mechanical impact usually starts with prolonged distress. Distress causes increased tension in the muscles, triggering the fight or flight response and faulty breathing. The tense muscles utilize more oxygen and produce more acid which in turn causes muscle ache and chronic fatigue.

Circulating ANP from the heart accelerates the process of fat burning and also promotes the production of omnipotent stem cells.

A study performed by Beldoch and his team at the Department of Psychology, Kent and Washington University, St. Louis showed a close association between atrium size and memory deficits. Insufficient release of ANP can accelerate heart failure and a decrease in the blood supply to the brain, resulting ultimately in poor memory.

Heart's Hormone Type B: BNP

The second mighty guardian of cardiovascular health is type B heart hormone. Its full name is the brain natriuretic peptide (BNP) because it was firstly identified in the brain by Sudoh T. at al.

Structure of the BNP

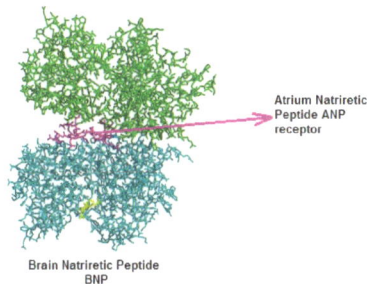

Atrium Natriretic Peptide ANP receptor

Brain Natriretic Peptide BNP

Figure 23 Displays the 3D structure of natriuretic peptide B (BNP) with ANP-receptor in purple colour
Wiki Commons , Public domain

The name of the second heart hormone may suggest that its origin is the brain. However, although BNP targets the brain, it is produced in the heart. The discovery of BNP was the second step in confirming the unimaginable intelligence of the heart. BNP is the chief hormone involved in heart/brain communication. It is released when the heart loses strength and does not supply the brain with sufficient blood and oxygen. BNP converts impulses that would otherwise harm the brain into benign or beneficial signals. It can dilate the brain's constricted network of blood vessels and also relieve spasms in the heart and brain. On publication of Sudoh's work, BNP became one of the most commonly used biomarkers when investigating a heart's functionality.

More recently, European molecular biologists have found that circulating BNP levels can indicate that the heart muscle, or myocardium, is hibernating. When the heart enters the hibernation process it puts the brain at risk. An elevated level of BNP indicates a need for improved oxygenation for both organs: the heart and brain. Measuring a patient's BNP level is very helpful in identifying heart or brain hibernation (more on hibernation later).

Interestingly, BNP levels are also associated with male and female sex hormones. Levels of progesterone, oestrogen and testosterone can stimulate or decrease the release of BNP as has been shown in the study performed by Passimo C. at al.

Heart's Hormone Type C: CNP

In 1998 Finnish researcher Dr. Virpi Tervonen and his team described the salmon natriuretic peptide, which is now confirmed as the C type heart hormone.

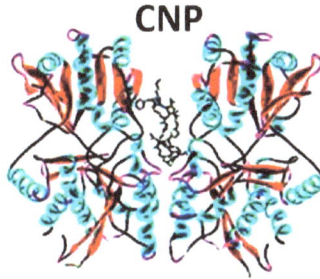

CNP

C Type Natriuretic Peptide

24 Molecular structure of the C-Type natriuretic peptide CNP
The Department of Physiology of The Institute of Arctic Medicine at the Oulu University, Finland

It is well established that a diet that includes salmon is beneficial for a healthy cardiovascular system. The C-type natriuretic peptide (CNP) is specifically related to the neuronal and autonomic functions of heart with its specialized nerves. CNP supports the correct functioning of the heart's electric conductive system and the heart's intelligence.

This type C heart hormone has a big impact on the heart's day/night rhythm and is one of the major factors supporting heart rate variability (HRV). An irregular or faster heartbeat in a resting position could be an indicator that the blood level of CNP is low. Decreased levels of CNP can impede the dissolving of blood clots and lead to blocking of small blood vessels.

Interestingly CNP helps in resolving blood clots and supports smooth, effective blood flow in coronary arteries.

The protective release of the C type heart hormone takes place in many heart rhythm disorders:

- CNP down-regulates the heart's rhythm, to protect the heart muscle from overstimulation.

- Conversely, a slow heartbeat indicates that the electrical system of the heart needs more regeneration and so CNP circulation will increase
- CNP also manages the levels of minerals necessary for heart health, such as Potassium, Magnesium and Sodium. Sometimes an irregular heartbeat can be caused by lack of Potassium, which supports heart muscle contraction. But an oversupply of Magnesium contributes to heart rate irregularities that can lead to sudden cardiac death.

Exercise naturally accelerates the heartbeat. Intense, forced breathing and respiratory muscle training can also bring about an elevated heart rate. Some natural spices and ingredients such as ginger or galangal can be also used as rhythm stimulating agents. An increased intake of natural (and not coloured) salmon in the diet may help to restore the electrical balance of the heart.

Sports people and professional athletes train not only their muscles but also their hearts. This training enables them to release more CNP as and when the body needs it. The intensive training they do trains their hearts to increase the volume of blood ejected with every heartbeat. So an athlete's heart delivers the same blood supply to their hard-working internal organs and muscles with fewer heartbeats.

CNP supports the heart muscle's regeneration and stimulates heart cells to produce more powerful growth factors (GFs). Nowadays, the GFs contained in platelet rich plasma (PRP) injections became very popular. PRP is an extract of the own blood containing small amount of stem cells, growth factors (GFs) and also CNP. GFs are widely used for facial skin regeneration, correcting wrinkles and gum regeneration. The injection of PRP directly into the joints can even accelerate the renewal of cartilage and bones.

CNP also plays an important role in healing the heart muscle itself. CNP prevents small scars building, which can occur when hibernation exists for a longer time.

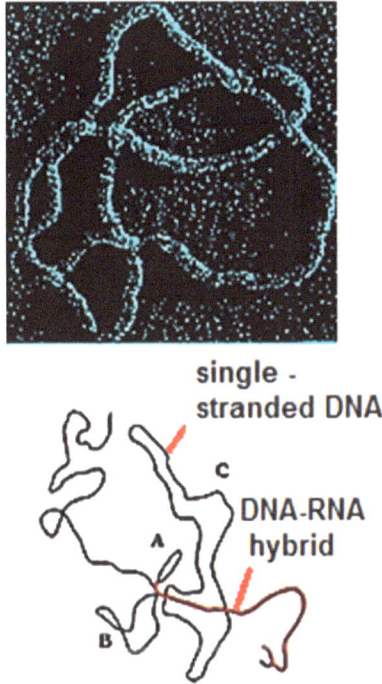

single -
stranded DNA

DNA-RNA
hybrid

Figure 25 The image of the knotted DNA
.The mechanism of self-entanglement is
a genetic attempt to repair the corrupted
DNA
*Figure 25 The image is credited to
N.Cozarelli*

During hibernation, the heart's cells are not sacrificed, they stay viable in a survival mode cause by low oxygenation, but their DNA may get knotted. The strands get twisted in the process of read-out of genetic information. It is kind of DNA impairment and the C type of the heart hormone CNP and it can support the process of the unknotting loops of DNA.

Such processes can be essential for the corrections in DNA in the hibernating cell of heart muscle so that the read out of the information is correct. The correct decoding of instructions for making proteins occurs in the process of transcription of information from the DNA to RNA and splicing of the genes from pre-mRNA (messenger RNA). The mRNA brings the message to the protein factory in the heart's cell. This is how the cell convert DNA into working proteins. Each of these phenomena – heart hibernation, the knotting of DNA, and at the edge of dying heart cells with the ongoing regeneration deliver powerful impulses to the brain and can cause anxiety in the impacted mind.

For 15 years, Dr Phillip A. Sharp's secretary kept a bottle of champagne refrigerated and ready for the special day her boss at the Massachusetts Institute of Technology won a Nobel Prize. He was rewarded in 1993 with the Nobel Prize in physiology or medicine for his discovery of "split genes." Splicing of the genes is the process in that from the copy of the copied RNA, the noncoding parts are cut out (exons) in order to connect the coding copied DNA parts. Dr Sharp found that this process of genes' splicing is the most common type of gene structure change in higher organisms, including humans. Sharp's discovery highlighted the knotting of DNA in cells before they undergo a controlled death process which helps maintain the integrity of the human body.

In 2016 He Wang and colleagues provided the first full profile of how DNA initiates the growth of the heart from embryonic beginnings to the mature adult heart. Your DNA determines the strategies your body will use to restore its damaged heart. The discovery of split genes confirms that the human body writes "the story of its life" continuously, from its very beginning to its maturity.

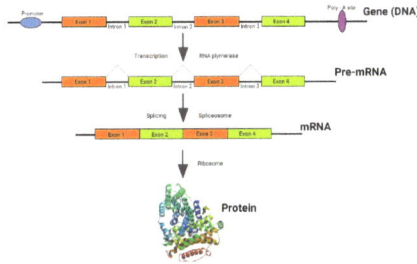

Figure 26 Transcription the information from the DNA to RNA and splicing of the genes from pre-mRNA (messenger RNA)
Wikipedia Commons by Ganeshmanohar

Heart's Hormone Type D: DNP

Dendroaspis natriuretic peptide (DNP) is the most recently discovered heart hormone. DNP opens small blood vessels and prevents the development of "micro clots". Scientists estimate that, if all of the veins and arteries in a human body were strung together, they would extend to 98,000 km in length, which is long enough to cause some elements of our blood to get stuck here and there in microcirculation on a daily basis.

With such a vast network of blood vessels it is understandable that micro blood clots are developing and being cleared away all the time. This is a natural process. Blood clotting is controlled through many blood related factors. However, DNP is a powerful agent in keeping the circulation free from blood clots and in preventing heart attacks and micro-strokes.

DNP supports smooth blood circulation, even in difficult conditions such as long-lasting stress or dehydration, or an extremely low level of oxygen. It keeps the blood fluid even under extremely dry weather conditions.

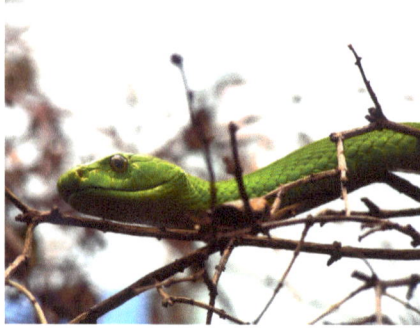

Figure 27 Eastern green mamba, native to the coastal regions of southern East Africa
Wiki Commons

DNP was first isolated from the venom of the green mamba, a highly venomous African snake of the genus Dendroaspis. In 1999 an almost identical hormone was identified in the human heart by Schweitz H. et al. It was named the dendroaspis natriuretic peptide (DNP). Toxicologists know that the bite of a green mamba causes major bleeding to internal organs resulting in death. Damage occurs because the snake's venom is 100 times stronger than human DNP, and it will completely stop the process of blood clotting in humans. So, the small amounts of DNP issued by the heart are essential in keeping blood flowing smoothly and keeping clots at bay. But too much of this stuff – as delivered from a mamba snake bite – will kill you.

Additionally, DNP activates the gut and stomach's movements known as peristalsis which is essential for good digestion and it facilitates the intake of water for the better functioning of the heart. The heart/small intestine connection is a part of traditional Chinese medicine framework, recognizing the small intestine as the most important functional partner of the heart..

Furthermore, DNP also supports the production of anti-inflammatory agents acting in our body similar to aspirin.

4. The Heart, the Brain and the Lungs

The Heart-Brain Connection

The discovery of the first heart hormone, ANP, in 1980 led to the development of a new discipline known as neurocardiology which studies brain/heart communication. Specifically, the heart and brain deal with massive amounts of data collected from all over the body. The cooperation of these two vital organs brings about the intelligent prioritisation of information and Adenosine plays a major role in this process.

Adenosine, the Heart's Regulatory Hormone and a Neurotransmitter

Novartis is researching adenosine, a hormone mediator that is very important for heart/brain interaction, general energy production and the circadian rhythm. Adenosine is one of the most intriguing human hormones. It is present in every cell and in especially large amounts in the heart and brain.

Depending on whether it is in the brain or heart, adenosine can have quite opposite effects; it can stimulate the heart but, as the day progresses, it also calms the brain, causing evening tiredness and the urge to rest.

It regulates the heartbeat and tunes the sleep/wake rhythm of the internal clock. Adenosine is also active in the maintenance of body temperature, blood pH, and the balance of minerals and water. It supports the elimination of toxins.

Adenosine triggers the CLOCK gene. Using a complex dialogue between metabolism, circadian rhythm and physiological functions, it enables our bodies to exploit the geophysical environment during the day and to rest and recover at night. We cannot expend energy without having a break. We need rest and good sleep for renewal and regeneration. This circadian cycle is a natural process. Adenosine causes an instant improvement in the blood supply within coronary circulation. This special effect of adenosine has been extensively studied for therapeutic and diagnostic purposes. The adenosine molecule has a striking similarity to caffeine, which explains why caffeine is so good at keeping us alert.

A special type of adenosine receptor, the A2A, is an important factor for inflammatory brain responses. The A2A receptor, discovered in 2012, controls the movement of immune cells across the blood-brain barrier. In light of this, adenosine may hold the key to treating multiple sclerosis (MS), a neuro-inflammatory disease of the central nervous system.

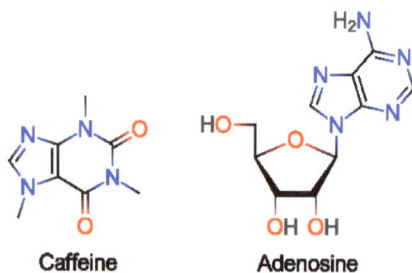

Caffeine   Adenosine

Figure 28 The structural similarity between Caffeine and Adenosine. It is the reason why the caffeine keeps us alert and vigilant
Wikipedia Commons No machine-readable source provided

The structural similarity between Caffeine and Adenosine. It is the reason why the caffeine keeps us alert and vigilant.

5. Challenges to the Human Heart

The world is facing an urgent, multifaceted heart health crisis. Recent advances and discoveries in cardiology and neuroscience indicate that the time is right to apply this cutting-edge research to create a response to the global cardio-pandemic.

The inability of contemporary medicine to arrest the global decline in heart health has shaken the conventional medical approach right to the core. Out-dated models of health – and heart health in particular –

do not reflect the complexity, dynamics and pace of the modern world. Contemporary medical business models are based on death-related and illness-centred stereotypes. There is no place in the current paradigm for the intelligence of the heart. The importance of the breathing mechanism and proper oxygenation of the body are not considered.

Prevailing profit-oriented business models are not focused on the interconnection between our inner and outer worlds, and not at all on the electromagnetic morphogenetic body field. Neither society nor individuals are treated holistically. Our symptoms, the bodily warning signs, do not match our changed life circumstances. The body is not mapped adequately in our awareness and not included in the development of individual consciousness.

The risk of death from cardiac catheterization, a diagnostic procedure, has been demonstrated at 0.11%. It means that 1 out of every one thousand patients undergoing this diagnostic procedure, dies. By 2.4 million diagnostic procedures performed in the USA, Europe and Asia together means that 2,400 patients died in 2018 during their cardiac diagnostics. These tragic statistics point to a very strong need for holistic and personalised heart health programs. The rising number of fatal heart incidents demands answers on a personal and global scale.

The heart may form coronary artery blockages or coronary spasms, and often enters a state of unpredictable hibernation to protect the heart's cells from immediate death. Sometimes it scrambles into erratic heart beats which, all of a sudden, can greatly diminish our health and wellness.

Sudden Death

The human heart can fail to ward off a heart attack, even after 30 or 40 years of biased performance. It can sometimes fall into uncoordinated, chaotic rhythm such as atrial fibrillation or palpitations. And sometimes a regular heart rhythm is interrupted by premature ventricular beats or a series of abnormal heart beats.

All these incidents produce a turbulent vortex flow in the left chamber of the heart. The vortex flow in the heart chambers can cause dizziness in the brain, discomfort in the chest, heart palpitations or even cause a person to faint.

In the worst case, the chaotic rhythm can end in a serious condition called ventricular tachycardia or ventricular fibrillation. This sometimes is called the "dance of death", because the heart races with a speed of 300 - 400 hundred insufficient, weak beats per minute around the baseline. It can cut the blood supply to the brain and cause sudden death. This happens before another regular heartbeat can interrupt it or before support from outside can restore the regular heart rhythm.

This life threatening sequence of chaotic cardiac rhythm can be lethal within seconds or a few minutes. Worldwide, 17 million, mostly young, people die from sudden cardiac death or sudden unexplained death every year. Sudden cardiac death affects not only mature adults in their forties and fifties, but rapidly increasing number of young, physically fit people, who suffer unexpected heart attacks. Athletes and people without noticeable cardiac risk can also be affected.

Hibernation: The Intelligent Heart's Protective Mechanism

The heart's ultimate protective mechanism is "hibernating myocardium", which is a stunning example of the heart's innate intelligence.

In 1989 the distinguished professor S. Rahimtoola from Harvard University discovered that, when the blood flow to the heart muscle is reduced, the heart can detect this and respond by putting some of its muscles to "sleep". Normally when blood flow to a part of the body is cut off or significantly reduced, the tissue in the area just will die, due to lack of oxygen and other nutrients. But the heart is different. It can temporarily shut down non-critical areas of itself so that the remaining blood supply will be directed to and used by the muscles that are most essential to survival. This hibernation is the heart's protective response to an energy crisis caused by lack of oxygen. It can be caused by a blockage, an obstructing clot or a spasm of a coronary artery. Hibernating Myocardium is usually preceded by a period of stress and low oxygenation associated with shallow breathing.

Hibernating Myocardium

Hibernating Myocardium is a very common medical condition. We all experience it in a various forms several times during a lifespan.

Poor oxygenation of the heart tissue induces hibernation. The affected part of the heart stays vital (still alive) but in fact the cells are stunned through low oxygenation and they hover at the edge between life and death. They are waiting for a life-giving impulse, for augmentation of oxygenated blood to restart their normal function.

Sometimes, the person who is experiencing Hibernating Myocardium may assume that the symptoms and cardiovascular warning signs they are experiencing are the result of a change in the weather, or that symptoms have appeared because of a difficult personal or family situation. This could be right, but usually is not. The changing weather or increased family related confusions are affecting the heart and, if the heart were unable to enter the state of hibernation to protect itself, a heart attack would be imminent.

Protective hibernation negatively affects the major intelligent functions of the heart. Heart rate variability (HRV) is low; the measure of the strength of the heart muscles, the ejection fraction (EF) is also reduced. The *sleeping mode* of the heart can cause an irregular heartbeat, chest pain, chest discomfort with burning and even heart palpitations.

Hibernating Myocardium can be triggered by:

- insufficient, shallow breathing
- distressed lifestyle
- alcohol and exposure to other toxins and pollutants
- emotional trauma

- poor, disturbed sleep pattern
- informational overload of the cells
- side effects of medication

Due to the challenges of our modern life, the protective mode of the hibernating heart can be an on-going process with ups and downs. In fact, it affects the majority of our population, all ages, both genders and all ethnic groups without any exemption.

Turbulent Vortex Flow within the Heart

Hibernation temporarily protects the heart's tissue by granting heart cells immediate survival. However, the abnormal function of a hibernating area produces rigidity of the heart's wall, known as hypokinesia or akinesia. And this rigid heart wall causes a turbulent vortex flow, usually in the left heart chamber. The turbulence can reach the major blood vessels supplying our brain, which puts the brain under increasingly destructive forces.

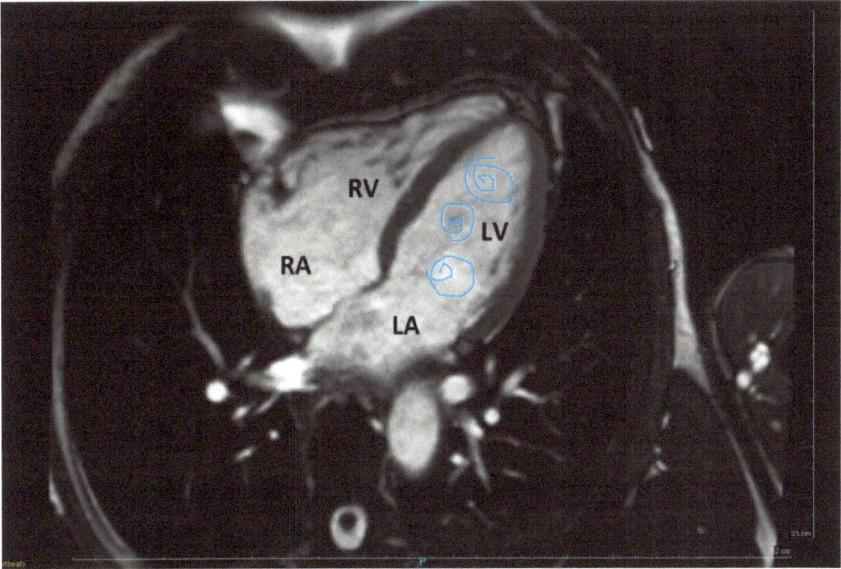

Figure 29 Vortex flow in all chambers of the heart captured during a MRI procedure. A turbulent flow is marked in the left ventricle (LV)
Own work

The vortex blood flow of the stressed, hibernating heart changes the harmonious pattern of the pulse and pressure waves. The smooth blood stream is altered and produces confusing and disturbing blood flow patterns. The picture shows magnetic resonance image in the left chamber with a turbulent flow.

The dark parts are related to the heart wall and the blood flow is coded with the grey scale. The vortex flow is coded with turquoise colour.

Hibernation can prevent an approaching heart attack. However due to the low oxygenation of the heart and brain, the spiral of negative effects in the heart can gain its momentum. It can impact the blueprint of health contained in the DNA. The turbulent vortex flow affects the functionality of the brain and mind.

The hibernation in the heart and the vortex flow that it produces can affect a person's experience and perception. This is a special kind of thinking and involves abnormal awareness, usually a narrowing of the scope of perception. The major internal organs are no longer properly synchronised and the mind is fully activated, searching for solutions. The conscious mind can be increasingly unfocused and cloudy. Very often insomnia and anxiety accompany the poor heart/brain cohesion. These symptoms are related to the brain but it is not really a brain condition. In fact, it is caused by the underlying dysfunctional state of *hibernating myocardium*. It is a real threat for the heart and brain cells, which are on the border between life and death.

Heart Attack Levels of Damage

If the oxygen supply does not improve, hibernation will progress and the chest pain (angina pectoris) will get worse. It can eventually cause a heart attack, involving damage to the heart muscle.

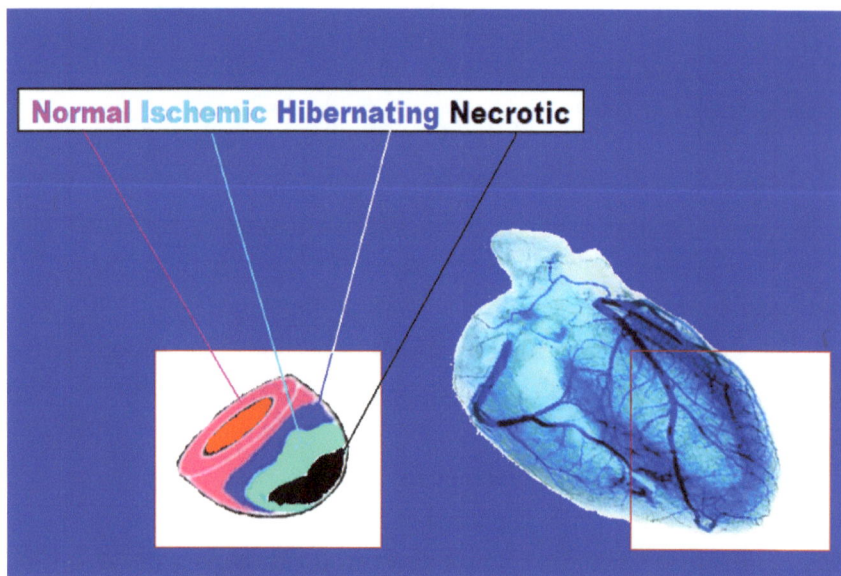

Figure 30 The progression of harm that is possible in a heart attack
Own work

The black zone symbolises the mostly irreversibly changed part of the heart (necrotic or dead tissue). If heart tissue is dying it means that the coronary vessel was totally blocked or closed by a spasm for a sufficient time e.g. hours. The cells' ability to survive can reach three to five hours from the occurrence of a heart attack. This period equals the time window for a cardiologist's emergency intervention. The red-rosé colour displays the normal heart tissue. The normal blood supply is coming from this area.

The turquoise colour indicates the surrounding zone, these cells are also at the edge of dying but this can be still reversed. This is known as the ischemic (poor blood supply and low oxygen level) zone. Under the ischemic condition the cells are able to stay alive for few hours more. Sometimes, the cells affected by ischemia can survive even a day or two days longer than the cells in the necrotic (dying) zone.

The deep blue zone correlates with the *hibernating myocardium*.

The blood supply is reduced and the normal functioning is restricted. The cells experience a shortage of oxygen but they can survive for longer. The intelligent heart can adapt to hibernation. Hibernation is a protective mechanism which can persist for weeks, months or even years. During this time, the heart's functions are at a lower metabolic rate but the human body can adapt to it. But over time we accept our limitations and the body stops its heart health restoring activities.

Sometimes this timeline of events can be classified incorrectly and seen as just the inevitable progress of aging. But in fact it is a malfunction of the heart which can be addressed.

Practical Actions to Prevent Hibernation and to Wake up the Hibernating Heart's Cells

The good news is that the *"sleeping mode"* of the heart can be prevented at its early stages by boosting the oxygen supply to the hibernating cells. Here's how:

- Be a knowledgeable Quantum Observer of your cardiovascular symptoms, recognizing the hibernation and its protective nature. More on this later.
- Increase your breathing capacity with regular respiratory muscle training.
- Do cardio training, to develop and train the heart to combat poor oxygenation and condition.
- Consider daily physical training and aerobic, oxygen dependent exercises such as Pilates, Yoga or Qi-gong
- Lead a healthy lifestyle and adequate nutrition, avoiding lectins and toxins such as alcohol.
- Try inhalation of air enriched with oxygen provided by a modern oxygen concentrator.
- Visit your GP on regular basis to manage any cardiovascular medication.
- Ask your GP about medication to augment coronary blood flow and be informed about their common side effects.
- In many Cardio related situations, an operation or medication can save your life, by reopening or relaxing the coronary vessel or increasing blood supply to affected areas of the heart. A heart attack can be aborted many times in course of one lifespan.

The development of portable oxygen concentrators is a new and modern approach. This machine directly separates oxygen and nitrogen via a system of mineral, molecular micro filters called Zeolite. Oxygen concentrators are considered safe for patients' use in their homes.

Home oxygen concentrators allow patients to utilize more oxygen and help to prolong the survival of the hibernating heart's cells in any emergency situation. Increased oxygen supports the respiratory muscle workload which increases the air volume intake with respiration.

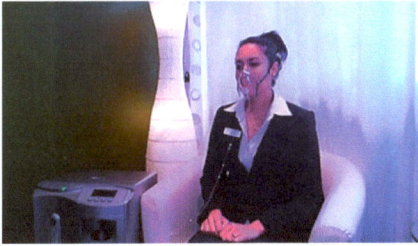

Figure 31 Patient with a portable oxygen concentrator
Own work

Portable oxygen concentrators help to improve exercise tolerance. An adequate oxygen supply during exercise allows you to exercise longer and to increase stamina. Visit your GP, a cardiologist or a lung specialist to find out if a portable oxygen concentrator will benefit you.

Coronary Circulation and Its Ability to Maintain Perfect Functionality in a Dynamic Balance

The heart is continuously building and resolving small clots in plaques or in narrow coronary microcirculation. The coronary system is building micro-blockages and mini-clots on a daily basis, and the body's clotting and immune systems steadily resolves them, keeping coronary circulation in balance.

Small clots can cause coronary blood flow to slow down, to stagnate or even to stop.

A blood clot has two components: a stable, organized blood clot called a thrombus. The building of the first part, the micro-clot is displayed at the image. The second part, which can be soft can at any time separate and to go with the blood stream. When a blood vessel is injured, tiny blood cells called platelets rush to the site. Then the platelets combine with circulating proteins and Calcium clump together in a cross-linked mesh of fibres to form a stable solid mass to fix the damage, the injury of the coronary vessel lining. This is the reason that the Calcium score in the performed CT scan of the heart can increase. A soft blood clot in a coronary vessel can grow very quickly, and can obstruct blood flow totally in as little as minutes or hours.

The process of building and dissolving a clot can sometimes stimulate the tiny muscles of the coronary vessel to produce a coronary spasm. The coronary vessels are at risk of these functional spasms when the plaque gets hot (inflamed through bacteria or viruses with a local temperature increase).

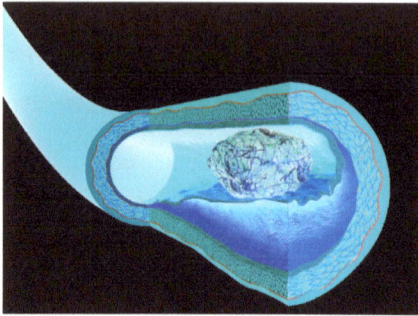

Figure 32 A blood clot. The platelets, the fibrin mesh and the immune system cells inside of a blood vessel
Wiki Commons by Blausen

The picture displays a blood clot. The platelets, the fibrin mesh and the immune system cells are the components building it. Clots form in an effort to prevent bleeding at the site of a micro-injury. Stagnation produces a vulnerable place of low resistance in the lining of the coronary vessel. This weak spot in the wall is susceptible to settlement of the further cholesterol crystals. Furthermore it attracts and feeds microbial invasion.

Blood clots pose an additional risk of a sudden coronary incident.

The best way to prevent any cardiovascular incident is to listen carefully to the messages from the intelligent heart. With the right understanding and practice individuals can sometimes restore a disturbed cardiovascular balance, and can limit symptoms at an early stage of their development.

Plaque

Plaque is defined as an injury in the lining of a blood vessel, caused by deposits of cholesterol and sharp calcium crystals, which is often infected by bugs or viruses. It starts usually with local damage of the vessel lining caused by toxins, increased acidity, mechanical stimuli, small, repeatedly occurring mechanical traumas or sedimentation of sharp cholesterol crystals. Prolonged circulating stress hormones such as adrenaline or noradrenaline can also produce small "bio-chemical scars" and can have a negative impact on the lining of the small coronary vessels.

Plaque is made up of fats, cholesterol, calcium and other substances in the blood. Calcium accumulates in a process called micro-calcification, and can make up to 30% of the plaque. Plaque can become infected with bacteria or viruses and this makes the plaque hot and vulnerable. The presence of plaque in a coronary blood vessel can restrict the flow of oxygen-rich blood to the muscles of the heart. The reactive plaque can trigger a coronary spasm triggering a blood clot that can cause a heart attack.

Plaque develops gradually over time and can narrow coronary arteries. Under favourable circumstances the effects of plaque can be mitigated through increased calcification. Calcification of plaque makes it cold and stable, and reduces the risk of heart attack.

A coronary calcium scan is the gold-standard non-invasive method for assessing the presence and risks of plaques in your coronary arteries. This heart scan is also known as a coronary calcium scan. It's a specialized X-ray that provides pictures of your heart that can help your doctor detect and measure the presence of calcium-containing plaque. The results of this test are reported as an Agatson score, named after the American cardiologist and celebrity doctor Arthur Agatson.

According to the *Australian Journal of General Practice* performed by Chua A. et al. your risk of heart attack or stroke increases along with your Agatson score:

However it should be remembered that calcification is the major, natural way for the body to mitigate the risks associated with vulnerable plaque within coronary arteries. The ability to calcify the vulnerable soft, reactive plaque is a healthy response of the body's self-organising system. Calcification is one of the intelligent actions of the heart itself.

As calcification increases, plaque becomes more solid and less vulnerable, which prevents it bursting and triggering a blood clot that can cause a heart attack. This healing process can cause a higher coronary calcium score which can be incorrectly interpreted as increased risk of heart attack or stroke.

A practical illustration of this fact is the case study of Elly. She underwent a coronary calcium scan in December 2012 and her score was 496 indicating a high risk because of the calcification in the left coronary artery, which added 354 points to the Agatson score. She has had several risk factors including smoking and high cholesterol, and decided to change her life style. Elly changed to a healthy diet and in the last four years she has practiced respiratory muscle training, Pranayama yoga and acupuncture to lower her stress levels.

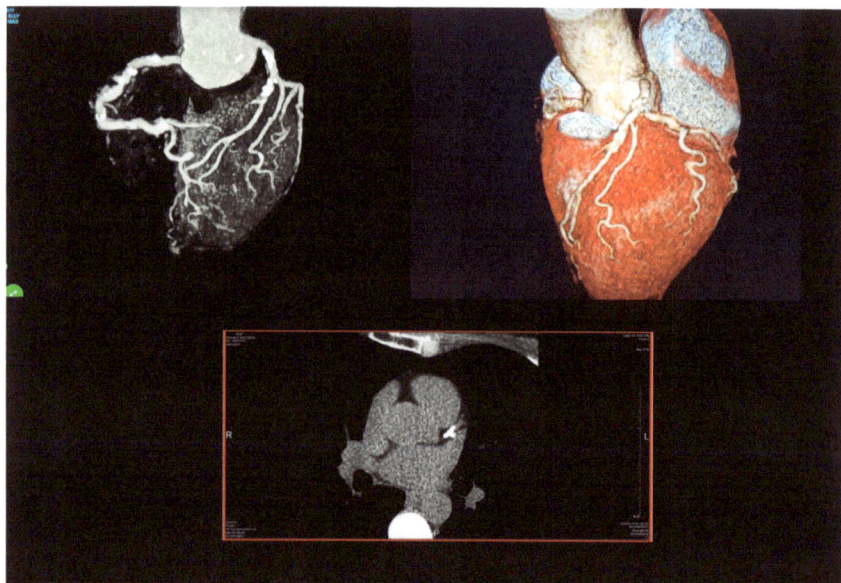

33. Elly's coronary calcium scan from 2012. Her calcium score was 496 bottom part of the picture The modern CT Coronary Angiography (CCTA) scan of Elly's heart in 2021—a more sophisticated technique, which can visualize the white calcium spots, and the course of coronary arteries and their plaques at the upper part of the picture
Own work. Courtesy Elly W.

Nine years later, in October 2021, Ellie underwent a more recent form of heart scan called CCTA, or Coronary Computed Tomography Angiography. This non-invasive procedure looks at the arteries that supply blood to your heart and can reveal vulnerable plaque. CCTA has been available for about a decade and about 26 million CCTA scans are performed globally each year.

The new scan showed an increase in calcified spots and Elly's Agatson score increased to 902 (up from 496). As a result, Elly was advised to be admitted to hospital for further diagnostics and eventually for a bypass surgery.

Elly was stunned by the results because she had spent years following a very healthy lifestyle.

Interestingly, the CCTA scan showed that the flow of blood in the coronary arteries was actually sufficient.

Elly decided to undergo a treadmill test with stress echocardiography, to assess the vitality and performance of her heart under strenuous exercise. The technicians were able to watch the beating heart at work while it was put under physical stress.

After the test, Elly's cardiologist reported that no disturbed movement of the heart walls and no ischemia (decreased blood supply to the heart muscles) were detected. Elly was reported to have an excellent exercise performance for her age. Elly could accelerate her heart and body metabolism to 12.5 MET metabolic units, where achieving an exercise workload of ≥10 METS predicts a very low risk of inducible ischemia. as it is evident from the study performed by Bourque J. M. at al.

In other words Elle was not at risk to develop angina pectoris or heart attack and continues her healthy life style today, including healthy diet, respiratory muscle training, yoga classes and medical acupuncture treatments. The case study suggests that an increasing calcium score may be considered indicative of the efficient healing of vulnerable, hot and reactive plaques in the coronary arteries.

This increase in plaque calcification in a patient who is healing is known as a paradox effect of statin therapy, and is associated with shrinking plaques as indicated by Consult QD in Plaque Paradox: *"Statins Increase Calcium in Atheromas Even as They Shrink Them. Not all coronary calcium is the same, analysis shows"* published in the Heart, Vascular and Thoracic Research of the Cleveland Clinic.

The scientific community is coming to recognise that calcification of the coronary arteries can be indicative of a curative effect on vulnerable, hot and reactive soft plaques as has been shown in the study performed by Iryna Dykun et al.

Situations Requiring Immediate Action

Heart dysfunction sometimes requires immediate action. If the symptoms do not stop, an ambulance is needed.

If you experience symptoms in the chest, do not assume it is heartburn, or stomach ache, indigestion or muscle pain. In 90 per cent of cases these cardio symptoms and warning signs come from the heart and must be addressed immediately. Assertive and knowledgeable action can be lifesaving.

Hibernating cells will survive longer if their oxygen supply is increased, but increasing oxygen is not so easy in the middle of a cardiovascular event. A good outcome depends on urgent, knowledgeable medical action. It is critically important that the patient and those in attendance understand the condition of the heart.

Whether the issue is with an ischaemic or hibernating zone, both have a chance to return to normal functionality when the blood and oxygen supply are quickly restored. Here are some vital steps for managing urgent cardiac symptoms:

1. This is an emergency. Every second counts.
2. Call an ambulance or see a doctor immediately.
3. Check the symptoms. Take note of: the character of breathing (rapid, slow, weak...), regularity of the heartbeat (consistent or irregular), pulse rate (beats per minute), and blood pressure, if possible.
4. Communicate the symptoms clearly to the ambulance despatcher or doctor.
5. Take a resting position and breathe slowly and deeply from the abdomen, in order to improve heart oxygenation

6. Check with the doctor or ambulance despatcher whether you should take an aspirin. This can help to resolve a blood clot, if that is the issue.

These steps may help the cells in the ischaemic and hibernating zones (the deep blue and turquoise areas) survive until the ambulance arrives. If the blood and oxygen supply do not increase, the cells in the threatened ischaemic zone will share the destiny of the cells in the necrotic (black zone) and will die too.

If these self-managed steps stop the symptoms it is a good sign. But if the actions do not ease the symptoms, you must call an ambulance immediately and follow the instructions of the ambulance despatcher and attending medical professionals. Once admitted to the emergency department, a full cardiovascular assessment will be done.

The cardiovascular system is adept at coping with arterial blockages. Even blockages up to 50% of the diameter of the vessel are usually well tolerated by most patients. However an additional spasm of the coronary vessel around the plaque can increase the existing blockage to 80% or 90% of the original diameter, and this can make the symptoms worse.

Treating coronary artery spasm

A specific cardio centred medication can help to release a coronary artery spasm. The most common medication in emergencies is nitro-glycerine, which can quickly relieve spasms of the coronary arteries. It is used to treat heart conditions, such as angina pectoris. Nitro-glycerine is administered preventatively, ahead of invasive procedures like a coronary angiography or an angioplasty. Nitro-glycerine acts to relax the special small muscles located inside and around coronary blood vessels. It triggers instant relaxation and prevents further narrowing of the arteries through a spasm, and at the same time prevents clots building.

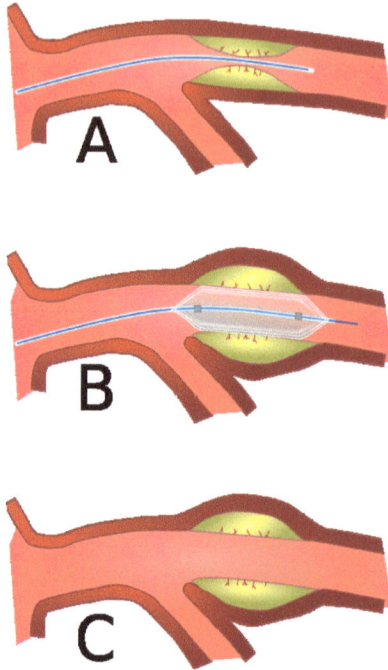

Figure 34 Coronary angioplasty, or percutaneous coronary intervention (PCI), is non-surgical procedure to treat narrowing of the coronary arteries with a balloon.
Wikipedia Commons by Schneepflug

The commonest invasive procedure to restore blood flow in a blocked coronary artery is coronary angioplasty. Coronary angioplasty needs to be performed in a hospital or in a specialized ambulatory unit. The procedure involves mechanically opening of the blocked vessel using a specially inflated angioplasty balloon. The first coronary angioplasty was successfully performed in 1977 by Dr Andreas Gruentzig, a German cardiologist working in Zurich, Switzerland.

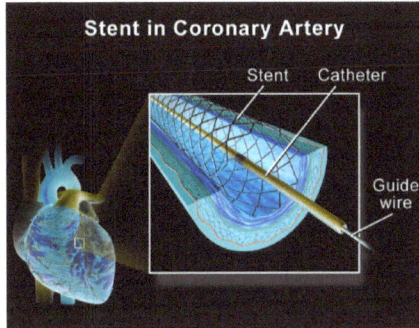

Figure 35 The picture on the left shows a coronary artery and the magnification shows the coronary vessel with the implanted stent.
Wiki Commons by BruceBlaus

Sometimes after a successful coronary angioplasty a stent (special scaffolding placed into the coronary vessel) is necessary to prevent the collapse of the dilated artery after coronary angioplasty. Once the hibernating myocardium is awakened and a spasm of a coronary artery is released, blood flow is restored and all is well again.

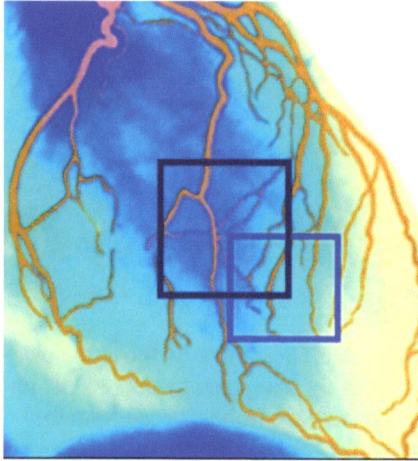

Figure 36 A color coded MRI scan of a
heart with restored coronary blood flow
after a successful coronary
angiography. The coronary vessels are
all open and supplying the heart muscle
Own work

Fortunately, there is no long lasting memory of such cardiovascular incidents. If the incident does not repeat within the next three weeks, the cellular memory is eradicated. The heart does not remember the previous symptoms, the chest pain, the chest discomfort, the shortness of breath and the accompanying anxiety. This is another powerful, protective mechanism of the intelligent heart. Otherwise, it would accumulate all the information of illness and never feel well again. After an incident of functional heart disorder it is a wonderful feeling to be healthy again. The intelligent heart, your best friend, does not remember the pain.

Junk DNA and the 7TM Receptors

If your grandfather and father suffered a heart attack, then you must act to avoid the same fate. It is an obligation to step up and come out of this negative deadly spiral. Anybody with a family history of cardiovascular disease has to conquer the curse of the generational genetic load.

It is possible to overwrite the old DNA program. This is the power of epigenetics.

Your insufficient health education, poor exercise level and unhealthy lifestyle all, at least partly, derive from the information passed down from your forebears.

If you don't step out of this toxic legacy, you will hand on the same heavy struggle to the next generation and will plant the same old negative seeds into the future.

An unhealthy lifestyle causes vital genes to be darkened in the process of DNA methylation. Methylation is a bio-chemical process that silences inactive places in the DNA.

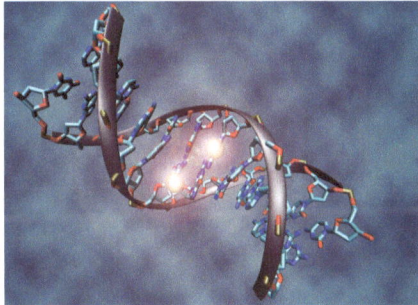

37 Representation of a DNA molecule that is methylated. The two white spheres represent methyl groups. A sequence of DNA
Wikipedia Commons by Christoph Bock

Seek wisdom; persevere in the will to find new knowledge in all areas of life. Find and seize all opportunities for good health.

The intelligent heart and body contain real and undiscovered treasures. Each of us is well equipped to rewrite junk DNA and to overcome our ancestors' imperfect DNA code, which becomes part of our inherited genes.

Correct Cardio functionality depends on 7TM receptors sensitivity. Junk DNA is the part of the genome that does not code for a protein and does not seem to serve any useful purpose. It constitutes about 98% of all DNA in humans. Susumu Ohno, a Japanese scientist in the early

1960s coined the term "junk DNA" published in "Biographical Memoirs, National Academy of Sciences", for the non-coding, inactive part of the human genome.

The human body is well equipped to sense and to respond to all cardio related symptoms. The 7Trans Membrane receptors, short the 7TM receptors inform the DNA about the impacts and actions at the cellular surface.

G proteins coupled with the 7TM receptors translate impulses into information and downstream the messages to the DNA. The genomic intelligence manifests our bodies in our 3D Reality and uses the communication with our mind to inform us about any bodily threats and symptoms/warning signs related to our internal organs, especially the heart and brain. The warning signs and symptoms will be then mapped in our brain and became part of our 3-D reality awareness. We need to be sensible enough to receive it, smart to decipher it and determined to take appropriate, preventative action.

The 7TM Receptors Have a Dish/Antenna for the Multilevel Communication

In 2005, Bruce Lipton led cutting edge research into the receptors. During his work on the topic of the Parkinson's disease, he was inspired by the incredible magnification of the electron microscope and he saw a special structure on the surface of the cell. It looked like an antenna. He described it and compared it to a satellite dish. In his bestselling book he stated that his discovery opens the way to a new understanding of human biology. Doing further research Bruce Lipton understood that the receptor is not only dealing with hormones and bio-chemicals but it has the ability to receive and react to invisible electromagnetic impulses like the TV antenna. This discovery initiated a paradigm change and revolutionized our medical concept of the cell communication.

The sensor of the cell, the 7TM Trans Membrane receptor at the cell surface, is quite special, like a bio-miniature mobile phone. The Intelligent Heart communication targets the 7TM in many ways. The 7TM receptor has seven loops (blades) going through the cell membrane. It looks like a dish or antenna. In the picture the 7TM receptor is marked in blue. Inside the receptor is a tiny crystal which is built up from 8 molecules of cholesterol (gold colour in the picture). The crystal responds to frequencies such as vibrations, sounds and electromagnetic waves. The cholesterol molecules in the receptor can be exchanged. The cholesterol molecules will be taken from blood to become a part of the 7TM receptors.

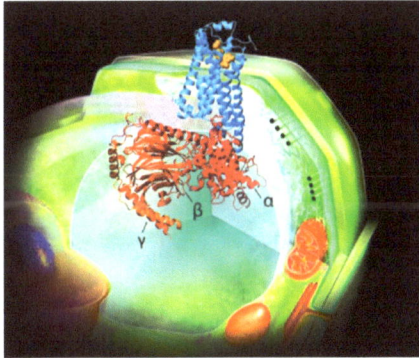

Figure 38 The G-Proteins are coloured red, orange and brown at the picture. They translate the impulses from the 7TM receptor outside the cell and transmit them to the cell's interior, to the DNA situated in the cell's nucleus
Own work

The G proteins act as sophisticated, molecular switches inside cells.

The seven loops (blades) of 7TM receptors are flexible and can change shape, taking on different forms according to what kind of impulse is approaching (hormonal, electromagnetic, acoustic). This process is called as conformation. The spatial change of the shape of the 7TM receptor is a signal for the receptor G coupled proteins to change their form and/or their position. This movement of the G proteins supports the 7TM receptor's change and its stabilization for the necessary time to activate a specific bio-chemical pathway. The created message is conveyed to the DNA. The genes know they are continuously supplied with the news from our internal world, from our environment and from the outer and inner space of man. The 7TM receptor is a multiple bio-tasker. It can:

- enact stimulations in our heart initiated by the heart's own hormoncs
- react to electromagnetic impulses and commands coming from our intelligent heart
- regulate water metabolism and energy production
- transform light into chemical reactions in our eyes to create our vision
- sense and monitor blood for sugar levels in the liver and pancreas, to produce adequate amounts of insulin
- answer to dopamine and serotonin in our brain to create either pleasant feelings or anxiety

So far more than 1,200 specific signalling pathways of 7TM receptors and coupled G proteins have been found. The multi-functionality of the 7TM receptor ranges from transforming light into bio-chemicals in the process of our vision to specific responses to the stress cascade, and to fine regulation of the blood cholesterol level. 7TM receptors respond to hormones such as oestrogen, progesterone and testosterone, and to bio-chemicals like dopamine, adrenaline or histamine. They receptors also respond to stimulation by small but relevant molecules like oxygen (O_2) or nitric oxide (NO). These small molecules enable the opening of constricted blood vessels and release vascular spasms in the coronary system. Oxygen is the major stimulating factor for the metabolism.

Adaptive down Regulation of the 7TM receptors Due to Informational Overload

The perfect function of the 7TM receptors fosters our vitality and intellectual wellness. G proteins are perfectly designed for precise communication with the heart, with the body and to transform the messages from the external environment. The capacity and capability of 7TM receptors to intake information and to send it into the cell interior is constantly challenged by the informational overload that defines the lifestyle of our modern digital society.

High and intense electromagnetic traffic at the membranes of the cells originate from personal computers, mobiles phones, computer screens, wifi routers and GPS devices. This electromagnetic impact can change the receptor status, can cause its translocation or even damage its function.

The human body is not designed to deal with digital coded information. The digital coding of frequencies with numbers (010101...) is the domain of modern, computerized technology. For example the global application of cloud computing generates a new category of health risks. The cloud is a highly compromised, condensed informational field surrounding us. The cloud contains a great amount data and electromagnetic energy in its perimeter. This energy is produced by the International Business Machines (IBM) virtual machines. The high energy wall is built in the cloud to defend access to information by cyber warriors and hackers. This energy can influence normal heart rhythm and the energy production of the cells. Our DNA can be corrupted by this unhealthy interference. It can disrupt the messaging cascade inside and outside of our cells and can deplete the 7TM receptors.

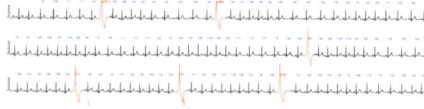

Figure 39 The heart creates analogue
frequency. It can be recorded as an ECG,
showing the electrical cyclic waves
originating from the heart. The black
cyclic ECG complexes are normal; the
red ones display abnormal heart beats
Own work

The human body works in analogue, in cycles and waves. It is not build by an artificial intelligence. It is not coded by numbers, not digitalized and not made virtual by man-made techniques. Even the brain produces nice, harmonious waves.

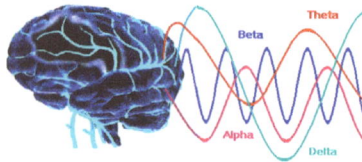

Figure 40 An electroencephalogram EEG
displays four forms of brain waves
known as beta, alpha, theta and delta,
which are different ranges of
frequencies
Own work

The heart, brain, gut and spinal fluid each generate a frequency. The healthy movement of spinal fluid has a dolphin-like movement. We build hormones and bio-chemicals and release them in waves throughout daily life. The human body has hormonal cycles. It regenerates and renews in a cycle of 21 days.

To change the underlying code of an inherited genetic expression, DNA needs to repeat the cycle of action, for example a sequence of bodily training, about 1,000 times. Internal contention, the conflict between analogue versus digital frequencies, and virtual realities all challenge real life. They overload our cells with information. This internal competition initiates the cells' protective response, but in the long term it leads to maladaptive actions.

Down Regulation of the 7TM Receptors

When the 7TM receptors, the analogue antennas of the cell, have to deal with a great amount of mixed digital and virtual frequencies over a long period, confusion ensues. At such times, the cells have to deal with higher levels of circulating stress hormones or to survive with low levels of oxygen.

The result is a protective response, reducing the sensibility of the cells, known as down regulation of the 7TM receptors. The 7TM receptors usually change their location (from outside, from the surface, to the inside of the cell) and therefore the process of downgrading the receptors is called translocation.

The overstimulated heart can become over-excited or develop a long QT-syndrome and cause heart rhythm disturbances, which in turn can end in a dangerous cardiac incident or death.

The good news is that the maladaptive process of downgrading the 7TM receptors is reversible.

There is only one way to upgrade the 7TM receptors: reduce the amount of circulating adrenaline and noradrenaline, and increase the oxygenation of the body.

Relaxation techniques, including medical acupuncture, professional massage, yoga stretching and qi-gong as described in the book of Dr Dyczynski J. "Inner eye" can help to recover these trans-located receptors. The task is to reduce the 7TM receptors' exposure to hormonal over-stimulation.

In the short term the application of a medication called β-Blockers[. These are some examples of generic and branded beta blockers: acebutolol hydrochloride (Sectral), atenolol (Tenormin), betaxolol hydrochloride (Kerlone),bisoprolol fumarate (Zebeta), carteolol hydrochloride (Cartrol), esmolol hydrochloride (Brevibloc), metoprolol (Lopressor,

Toprol XL), penbutolol sulfate (Levatol), nadolol (Corgard), nebivolol (Bystolic), pindolol (Visken), propranolol (Inderal, InnoPran),timolol maleate (Blocadren), sotalol hydrochloride (Betapace), carvedilol can bring temporary relief.

Beta-blockers are the drugs that bind to the part of the 7TM receptors connected to the stress cascade and therefore they block the binding of adrenaline and noradrenaline to these receptors. When the last receptors are blocked the body will assume that there is a complete stillness at the cell's surface and will relocate the receptors back to the surface. β-Blocker has some relevant side effects, but it works for the short term in clinical practice.

The medication applied for a short time - days or weeks - can help to reduce many of the issues associated with maladaptive downgrading the 7TM receptors, and restore the cells' sensitivity. Insensitive cells with downgraded 7TM receptors are less perceptive and less responsive to changes in the inner and outer space of man. This reduced sensibility is why some people fail to respond correctly to early symptoms originating from the heart and the cardiovascular system.

Insensitivity to gentle but alarming symptoms of the heart puts the cardiovascular system at an extra risk and will open the door to illness. A massive loss of cell sensitivity can even cause a silent heart attack (without any symptoms and warning signs) and can disrupt precious life.

The early self-detection of heart rhythm disturbances and identification of the heart as the origin of the chest pains is of great importance in the prevention of sudden cardiac death or sudden unexplained death.

The Impact of the Down Regulation of the7TM Receptors on Daily Life

The down regulation of 7TM receptors, resulting in a loss of sensors, affects the functions and the intelligence of your heart and disturbs the blood supply to the brain. An affected individual can feel disconnected from the breathing mechanism and separated from the outer and inner space of man. The pace of the breath slows down and becomes shallow, and the uptake of cholesterol is sluggish. The receptors do not take in enough molecules of cholesterol and circulating blood becomes thicker. The rising level of cholesterol in the blood leads to aggregation of molecules and to a build-up of cholesterol crystals outside the cells. In turn, these sharp crystals damage the lining of blood vessels in the brain and coronary system of the heart

Plaque

Plaque is sometimes called "hardening" or "clogging" of the coronary arteries). It is a micro-injury and a build-up of cholesterol and fatty deposits on the inner walls of the coronary arteries.

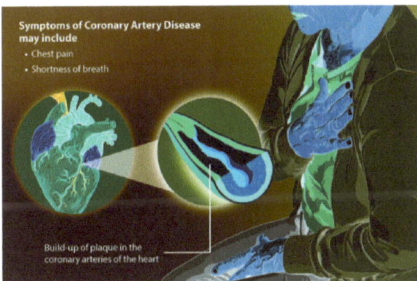

Figure 41 Plaque can restrict blood flow to the heart muscle by physically clogging the artery or by causing abnormal artery tone
Wikipedia Commons by Myupchar

Plaque can produce a small blood clot. It is displayed at the left side of the picture in red and purple. The growing clot makes further restriction of the function and can further narrow or completely close the vessel, and this will result in heart attack or stroke, depending on whether it manifests in the heart or brain. Plaque can also become "hot" through the invasion of bacteria. Increasing inflammation makes the plaque hotter. The inflammatory process can lead to a part of the "hot" plaque to break away and be carried along the blood stream to cause a stroke.

The intelligent heart and the cardiovascular system counteract the narrowing tendency in coronary vessels by increasing blood pressure. The heart pumps blood with more force to push it through the narrowed coronary vessel.

A loss of sensitivity in life is not only a failure of the heart. Prior to the loss of intelligent heart functions an affected individual experiences weakened breath. The breath gives life and sustains oxygen levels for use by all our tissues and internal organs.

Hibernating Myocardium

Shallow or distressed breathing will cause low oxygen levels in the body, especially in the heart tissue. When that happens, cellular intelligence can apply a protective mechanism to avoid a disaster and protect the cells from immediate death. In cardiology, this phenomenon is known as the *hibernating myocardium*. When the body is short of oxygen, part of the heart wall can enter into "sleeping mode", causing the wall to become rigid.

This reaction of the heart to reduced oxygenation was discovered by a distinguished Professor of Cardiology, S.H. Rahimtoola. He published his work in 1989, under the title "The Hibernating Myocardium" in the prestigious *American Heart Journal*.

The brain, affected by the hibernation of the heart muscle, can also develop a neuronal energy crisis resulting in brain tissue hibernation; otherwise the neuronal cells in the brain might die. Once an individual is affected by hibernating myocardium or by brain hibernation, vigilance and vitality diminish. The affected person is not focused, not sharp in perception and their short term memory declines. This is the next step of maladaptation to a shortage of oxygen. Hibernation in the brain is more serious; it is far worse than down regulated 7TM cell receptors and the loss of the cells' sensibility. Now the cells are at the point of life or death. If urgent action is not taken, a heart attack or stroke may follow. This is a life threatening situation that needs to be addressed with urgency. We humans need to address this, individually and globally, to win life back.

High Blood Pressure

A temporary rise in blood pressure to support our daily activities, according to mental and physical challenges, is something normal and natural. But chronic high blood pressure is a risk factor for heart attack, stroke and sudden cardiac death

Usually high blood pressure (BP) causes no pain. In the initial stage of its development the affected individual does not experience any cardiovascular symptoms. One symptom of incipient high BP is when blood vessels at the temples become more pronounced. Or a postnasal drip might indicate increased pressure inside the brain.

Alternatively, an activated stress reaction with the elevation of blood pressure can sometimes feel good. This nicely energized state is pleasant, but the energy comes from an inappropriate source. Many people assume that high BP is relatively harmless but elevated BP is a serious symptom of low oxygenation, usually related to chronic shallow breathing and many other factors causing long lasting cardio stress.

The elevation of BP is also a protective and compensating mechanism of the intelligent heart. The heart needs to adequately supply the whole body with oxygen, but O2 is lacking. This is a challenge for the heart and cardiovascular system. Elevated blood pressure initially accelerates blood circulation, to overcome reduced oxygenation in various parts of the body. When insufficient oxygenation lasts longer it hits the heart itself and affects the brain.

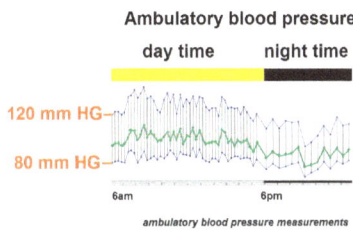

Figure 42 The blood pressure fluctuates throughout the day and night, but the average values are usually within the normal or optimal range
Own work

The two blue lines represent the systolic BP and diastolic blood pressure. The yellow zone is the day and the black zone is the night. The numeric values of the systolic BP are higher than the diastolic BP. The average blood pressure is displayed as the green line in the middle. In the night the BP goes down because of the deep sleep.

A longer lasting, elevated BP initiates the process of maladaptation towards factors that make you unwell: shallow breathing, physical inactivity, downgrading of the 7TM receptors and reduced oxygen for cellular breathing. At this stage the BP values are not only sporadically elevated they do not return to the normal baseline. BP is continuously too high, even in the resting position.

Furthermore elevated BP can cause excessive growth of the heart muscle. This occurs because, with narrower blood vessels, the heart now has to overcome much higher resistance and has to perform more work. The heart chambers can increase their size, and the atria or ventricle can enlarge.

The cause of permanent and elevated BP is poor synchronization between the heart and brain. This missing cooperation is linked to changes in intellectual wellness such as poor concentration, irritability and poor memory.

The Brain and Circulatory Systems

A closer look at the anatomy of nerves and blood vessels in the brain reveals their close relationship in our brains. The neurons and blood vessels of the brain's microcirculation build one inseparable cerebrovascular unit. It is almost impossible to distinguish nerves from blood vessels, as they are interwoven very closely. Whenever the brain is called upon to perform the firing neurons instantly receive more blood supply with fresh oxygen,

The blood vessels' instant response in the region of the increased brain activity is known as the neurovascular coupling.

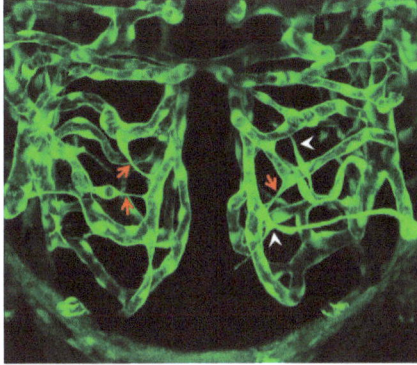

Figure 43 Developing brain blood
vessels, known as vasculature. The
small vessels include small, reactive
muscles opening wide to nerve
impulses. The vessel network
undergoes not only angiogenic
sprouting (arrowheads white), but also
extensive vessel pruning
Creative Commons by Sedwick

The neurovascular coupling can be depleted by long lasting high BP. Then the neurovascular coupling starts to be dysfunctional. At this stage the individual can already notice the first signs of lower energy and decreasing performance. The individual's usual dynamic behaviour and the accurate perception could be reduced by 60% or 70% or even more of the usual perception in the 3D space-time reality.

Ongoing, permanent elevated blood pressure is called hypertension. It signals an advanced stage of reduced oxygenation, causing a progressive downgrading of 7TM receptors and loss the cells' sensibility. This condition affects about a billion people worldwide.

Blood Pressure Lowering Medication

Hypertension, the permanent elevated blood pressure, is usually treated with prescribed medication. The alarming reality is that only about one-third of people who take medication for high BP are able to bring their blood pressure back into a safe zone. The remaining two-thirds are classified as the non-responders. This category also includes the non-compliant patients, who take their medication irregularly or in an inadequate dosage, and also patients taking other drugs that impede the effectiveness of the BP-lowering medication.

Many non-responders have downgraded 7TM receptors. Insufficient 7TM receptors make BP-lowering medications ineffective. Simply taking the prescribed medication too long can reduce its efficacy and render the patient a non-responder. Long term use can bring about a maladaptation to the drug and make it ineffective in lowering elevated BP. According to statistics two-third of patients with hypertension are exposed to the negative side effects of their prescribed drug.

The good news is that a personal genetic profile can reveal insensitivity to a specific drug. One's personal genetic make-up can be associated with either hyper- or hypo-sensitivity to a specific drug or its metabolites. Hypersensitivity can cause massive adverse reactions to a normal dosage of medication. Such effects include a massive drop in blood pressure with light headedness or even a tendency to fainting; or a massive allergic reaction; or a life threatening shock reaction. Another example of hypersensitivity can be strong Tinnitus in the course of the medication with a small dosage of Aspirin (ASA - Acetylsalicylic Acid). Similarly, a small dosage of 50 mg Aspirin taken to prevent blood clots can cause the patient to hear non-existing sounds, in reaction to salicylate hypersensitivity or toxicity.

In summary, elevated blood pressure over an extended period can accelerate plaque build-up in the coronary arteries, induce spasms, and can cause constriction of brain blood vessels and their hardening. High BP can produce a hypertrophic heart muscle, the long QT syndrome (prolonged relaxation of the heart muscle). These are only a few negative results of chronic elevated blood pressure. All these abnormalities put the affected individual at high risk for heart attack, stroke or even sudden cardiac death.

Atrial Fibrillation and High Blood Pressure Can Cause Memory Decline

It is common knowledge that atrial fibrillation (AF) carries a high risk of stroke. The illustration shows how a stroke can occur during atrial fibrillation. A blood clot (thrombus) can form in the left atrium of the heart. If a piece of the clot breaks off and travels to an artery in the brain, it can block blood flow through the artery. The illustration shows how a stroke can occur during atrial fibrillation. A blood clot (thrombus) can form in the left atrium of the heart. If a piece of the clot breaks off and travels to an artery in the brain, it can block blood flow through the artery. The lack of blood flow to the portion of the brain fed by the artery causes a stroke.

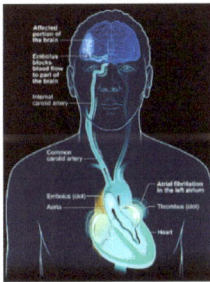

Figure 44 It is common knowledge that atrial fibrillation (AF) carries a high risk of stroke
Wikimedia Commons, Public domain

New research suggests that atrial fibrillation may put the heart and brain at increased risk of intellectual and memory decline, even if the patient was not diagnosed with a clinical stroke. In 2013 an evident link between atrial fibrillation and memory decline was found. The chaotic uncoordinated contraction waves and slower blood flow in the atrium can cause a stroke, as it is shown in this picture and confirm in the study performed by Wolf P. A. at al.

Evidence suggests that chronic high blood pressure significantly increases the risk of intellectual impairment, vascular dementia and Alzheimer's disease.

A good memory creates life force, the basic component for wellness.

For example, a study involving 2,505 patients with elevated blood pressure showed that 77% were more likely to develop dementia in comparison to the control group with normal systolic blood pressure below 120 mm Hg.

It seems that the intelligence of the heart is suppressed by fluctuating blood pressure. With chronic high blood pressure, the heart cannot supply the brain with sufficient fresh blood and oxygen, and both the heart and brain lose access to the field of memory.

"Broken Heart Syndrome"

Sometimes even the heart's resilience and intelligence cannot prevent the heart being literally broken. Broken heart syndrome was originally called *takotsubo* cardiomyopathy because the left ventricle takes on the shape of a *takotsubo*, a Japanese trap used to catch octopi in the study presented by Japanese researchers led by Akashi Y.

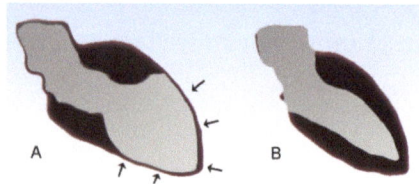

Figure 45 In a "broken heart", the left ventricle takes on the shape of a takotsubo, a Japanese trap used to catch octopi.
Wik Commons by J. Heuser

Broken heart syndrome feels like a heart attack, with typical chest pain and dizziness. Overwhelming stress disrupts the usual mode of abdominal breathing, causing poor oxygenation, which deepens the energetic crisis and the reduction in the supply of oxygenated blood. However the hallmark of a heart attack - the blockage of coronary arteries - is missing.

A functional spasm of a coronary artery can be a factor in broken heart syndrome, which temporarily reduces the blood supply to the affected region. After a while this spasm will resolve and the coronary artery will return to full functionality. Research suggests that up to 5%

of women evaluated for a heart attack actually have "broken heart syndrome". It has been recently reported that it may go largely unrecognized.

Chemical Exposure

Many of us are exposed to the gender specific side effects of medication. Our gene expression changes, due to increasing exposure to air pollution, and to chemicals and preservatives in food. Each of us young and old needs to deal with chemical exposure and to upgrade our 7TM receptors.

Medication

Our modern lifestyle, based on existing urban culture, lack of exercise, and insufficient oxygenation leads to increasing, uncontrolled self-medication, including caffeine and alcohol.

Electromagnetic Fields

The interference of 21st century electromagnetic fields disturbing the heart is mostly man-made. Urbanization and the 4th industrial revolution of the digital age produce innumerable, identifiable risks for health, including:

- insensitivity through downgrading of the 7TM receptors,
- premature degeneration,
- poor physical and intellectual wellness,
- susceptibility to accidents and injuries.

We are exposed to the impact of big data, 4G and 5G networks for mobile phones with the transmission towers placed every 300 meters from each other, and computational power. And 24/7 connectivity takes its toll on human health. Everyone has to deal with new forms of human-/computer/machine interaction, artificial intelligence, with augmented reality, with continuous improvements in transferring digital instructions to the physical world, robotics and 3D printing in the home and in medicine, nanotechnology in drugs delivery, new biotechnologies, sophisticated business models and internet dependency. All these technological advancements increasingly expose humans to the external Electromagnetic Field (EMF) and high energy radiofrequencies (RFs).

Some evaluations have been made concerning the strength of the electromagnetic power of the human heart. One of the estimates delivers an interesting comparison. It states that the electromagnetic field of the heart has 1/1000 of the power of the earth's electromagnetic field. It seems to be impossible from our first impression, because the earth is so vast. It becomes more understandable when you consider that only the superficial layer of the earth has an electromagnetic field. The deeper layers of the earth are rapidly losing their electromagnetic strength due to extremely high temperatures inside of our planet.

Further analysis of electromagnetic fields and the human body can lead to electromagnetic healing hands. This practical, empirical wisdom was gathered over the course of centuries. It considers that the electromagnetic field of the hands used for purposes of healing is very strong.

Intentionally applied hands for the purpose of healing can develop a magnetic field that is 1,000 times stronger than the field created by the heart. Therefore healing hands may be able to generate an electromagnetic field which is comparable to the electromagnetic field of the entire Earth.

The Earth's Electromagnetic Field: Schumann Resonance

The Schumann resonance represents the frequency of the Earth's electromagnetic field. It has always had stable electromagnetic vibrations at 7.83 Hz, with few variations since 1952. But in June 2014 there was a significant change. The Schumann resonance showed a sudden increase in activity from 8.5 Hz to 16.5 Hz.

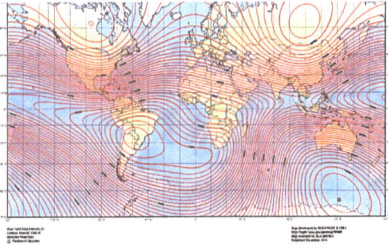

Figure 46 Map of the electromagnetic field of the Earth, Wikipedia
https://en.wikipedia.org/wiki/ File:World_Magnetic_Field_2015.pdf

Researchers were alarmed at these values, something that had never been recorded before. More recently, other peaks have been detected, increasing the planet's frequency to more than 30 Hz. This may explain the strange feeling for time flow. It seems to be that time is passing more quickly and this could be linked to the excess speed of Schumann resonance, which makes us feel a 24-hour period as if it were approximately 16 hours http://www.ultimatescience.org/frequency-electromagnetic-field-planet-earth-changing/.

Recent findings suggest that mobile phone networks as well as the processing power of human brains can affect the structure and the strength of the electromagnetic field of the Earth in the sudy made by Small G.W at al.

A minimum intensity occurs in the South Atlantic Anomaly over South America, while there are strong electromagnetic fields over northern Canada, Siberia, the coast of Antarctica and Australia.

Nutrition

The world population is moving to unhealthy nutrition choices. As a result, our modern lifestyle produces borderline hypertension, diabetes mellitus, obesity, heart attacks, strokes and 17 million lethal outcomes annually from sudden cardiac death SCD.

6. How Health is Overpowered by Illness

Electromagnetism

The first protective shield of the human body is electromagnetic. Gentle electrical current is everywhere in your body, caused by chemical reactions that occur as part of normal bodily functions, even in the absence of external electromagnetic fields. All your muscles, for example, are activated by electrical currents. Your nerves relay signals by transmitting electric impulses. All biochemical reactions, from digestion to brain activities, are a function of the rearrangement of energized particles. Your heart is highly electrically active, and you can see this activity with the help of an electrocardiogram (ECG).

Your Skin

The skin constitutes the second layer of protection of the body in 3D space-time. Your body is exposed to the outside environment in places like the nose, mouth and throat. In these places, instead of skin there is a special lining producing "mucosa", a thick protective fluid. This mucous membrane separates the intelligent, healthy information inside your body from the destructive power of illness residing outside.

The skin and the mucosa are wonderful protectors. They are a protective membrane between your 3D space-time manifested body and the electromagnetic 5th dimension outside of the body.

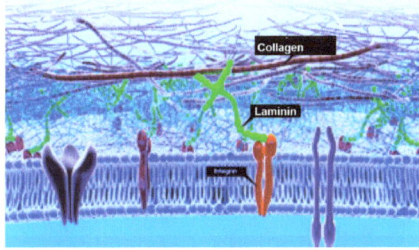

Figure 47 Skin is built from powerful,
resilient layers of collagen, laminin and
integrin. It separates the bio-universe
inside from the vast universe outside
Credit to Biolamina

When the destructive information of illness finds an entry point, a gap, firstly in the electromagnetic shield of your body, it will settle in the skin and cause a disorder. It can enter your body and overcome your vitality and immunity. If the destructive powers are strong enough it can break through the natural membranes of the skin and operate inside the body, making it much harder to cure.

Any illness can be reversed. Please embrace this fact with certainty.

The negatively charged information associated with illness is entangled with the intelligent health information found in the electromagnetic 5th dimension. Get your thoughts right, with the right intention, and the power of quantum healing can begin. This is the probability approach of medical physics the 21st century. Once awakened and supported through the knowledgeable actions of a skilled QO it will reach the level of singularity. The singularity as an autonomous process will cause an "explosion of the health" and the disease will leave the 3D space-time reality of the body. It will return to the invisible electromagnetic fabric of the Universe where it came from.

7. Diagnostics

Heart Rate Variability (HRV)

HRV is a very simple but sensitive measure of heart health. It is based on recordings of the electrocardiogram (ECG) reflecting the body's electromagnetic field. The heart constantly generates electricity and a strong electromagnetic field. A 2-minute ECG can generate a colourful Cardio Image of your heart and its present state of health. It will indicate subtle changes in the heart's action caused by elevated stress levels and changes in the blood supply to the heart. The stress level will be measured as Cardio Stress Index (CSI) in the range from 0 to 100% with an innovative heart screening technique using as visual signalling the traffic lights coding.

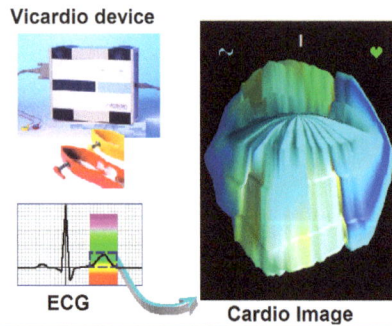

Vicardio device

ECG

Cardio Image

Figure 48 A small portable device for
registration of ECG and HRV
*Own work with extract from Energy-Lab
Technologies, Hamburg, Germany*

This small portable device Energy-Lab Technologies, 20095 Hamburg, Germany creates a dynamic window into essential cardiovascular functions and it is an evidence based tool to assess the heart/brain interactions, the dynamism of breathing mechanism and the levels of hormonal activity.

An example of a short term ECG and HRV recording in colors as a Cardio Image is displayed at the picture above. It codes the ECG and

HRV readings in colours and generates a pattern known as a Cardio Image within 2 minutes. It creates a dynamic window to assess essential cardiovascular functions, and indicates the changes caused by elevated stress levels and alterations of the blood supply to the heart itself. Any deviations from the exact timing of the electric potentials will be also recorded. An ideal heart portrait image is coded with blue and green colours. The Cardio Image will also indicate changes of the electric potentials and their exact timing, and it will show any abnormalities in the blood supply to the heart.

The HRV program also calculates and displays the individual's stress level, expressed as the Cardio Stress Index, or CSI. The individual's distribution of the three HRV frequencies is rendered as a pie chart showing the share of these frequencies. The distribution of three frequencies of HRV related to breathing/lung function, heart/brain interactions and hormonal/immune system activity.

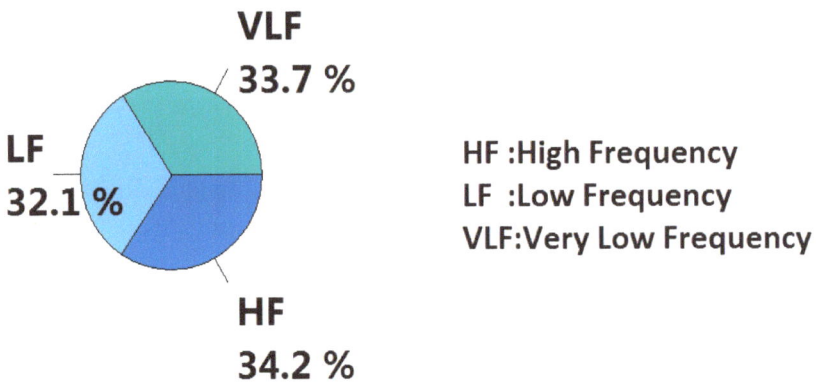

VLF
33.7 %

LF
32.1 %

HF :High Frequency
LF :Low Frequency
VLF:Very Low Frequency

HF
34.2 %

Figure 49 A normal distribution of three frequencies of HRV related to breathing/lung function, heart/brain interactions and hormonal/immune system activity.
Own work

- The first of the measured HRV components is the high frequency (HF), which is coloured in deep blue. It reflects mainly the function of the lungs and the level of the body's oxygenation

- The second HRV component is the low frequency (LF) colored as bright blue. It expresses mostly the heart functions. It also allows the estimation of brain/heart cohesion and coordination
- The third HRV component, the very low frequency (VLF) (displayed in green colour) is an extremely sensitive measurement. It acts as if the subtle release of hormones and bio-chemicals is a gentle sound in the body and can be recorded

VLF- is the frequency below ⁽0.04 Hz
LF - is the frequency from 0.04 to 0.15 Hz
H F - is the frequency from 0.15 to 0.40 Hz

Heart Frequencies

Three frequencies are literally "gentle sounds" originating from the specific functions of the body. The high frequency (HF) reflects the lung/breathing mechanism and the oxygenation of our body. The low frequency (LF) mirrors the heart functions and its cooperation with the brain. The very low frequency (VLF) relates to the hormonal system including the actions of the immune and defence system. The software displays the percentage of their distribution in an individual pie diagram. In ideal situation all three fields are equal like the well-known Mercedes star.

Case Study: Excess Stress

Let's consider a case study – a woman in a stressful situation. She presented with superficial breathing and chest tightness. She complained about sporadic burning pain in the middle of the chest, behind the breastbone. And she had a disturbed sleep pattern, accompanied by a high level of anxiety.

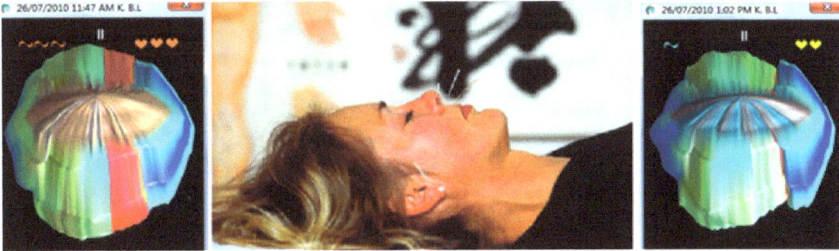

Figure 50 The cardio stress index (CSI), the Cardio Image on the left side was increased with 56%. The increased stress level is displayed as the brown coloration at the core, the "lead" of the Heart Image. The redness on the left could be related to a hibernation of a small heart area. On the right side of the image almost a normalization of the Cardio Image after acupuncture and respiratory muscle training
Own work

The cardio stress index (CSI), the image on the left side was measured at 56%, which was far above acceptable values (normally lower than 20%). The increased stress level is displayed as the brown coloration at the core, the "lead" of the heart portrait image. The redness on the left side of the picture indicated an area of the heart muscle with a low local functionality due to diminished blood supply and a lack of oxygen. It may be considered as a state of the heart's hibernation. The second cardio check from the same patient was recorded 1 hour and 15 minutes later, after an intense respiratory muscle training and medical acupuncture.

The relevant changes in colours of the Cardio Image confirm the normalization of the blood supply and a reduction of the Cardio Stress Index (CSI) from 56% to 20%.

In the prevention of sudden cardiac death (SCD), the most important is the measurement of the QT time interval. The QT time interval indicates how long needs the heart muscle to recharge between beats In long QT syndrome, your heart muscle takes longer than normal to recharge between beats. Too long relaxation of the heart muscle will produce Long QT Syndrome which constitutes a specific risk for sudden cardiac death.

Heart Rate Variability Indicates the Human Heart Perfect Function

Research conducted at The HeartMath Institute in California, USA has significantly advanced our understanding of heart-brain interactions. Their advanced research confirmed the importance of taking account of heart rate variability (HRV) in modern medical training, in cardiology and in sport medicine. The HeartMath Institute found that HRV accurately reflects the intelligence of the human heart. Heart interactions with the brain are known as coherence. HRV indeed visualizes the heart's responses to rapid alterations in mental state.

The external environment and bodily transformations on demand influence the HRV pattern. Heart rate variability indicates the flexibility of the heart's rhythm in adaptations to distress and the new, even utmost strange external conditions.

In their HRV research a team of researchers led by Dr. Rollin Mc-Craty achieved major breakthroughs in psycho-physiology, neurocardiology and biophysics. They enriched and simplified the science of the heart. In 1991 McCraty's team discovered the heart's unique nervous system. This neuronal system governs energy production, supply and distribution, and it is fully independent of the brain.

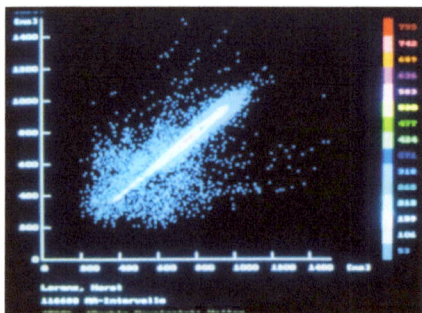

Figure 51 Twenty four hours registration of HRV
Own work

Heart rate variability is a key marker that gives us a valuable insight into the individual's stress level and their heart's intelligence. HRV reflects heart/brain functions, oxygenation, breathing and hormonal activities. HRV is evidence-based and is commonly used to monitor wellness and athletic fitness. HRV is helpful in assessing the brain's blood supply and its coordination with our intelligent heart functions, and the effectiveness of the respiratory muscles training RMT.

In the image above you can see a record of 24 hours of HRV. A good, working, intelligent heart function can be recognized as a regular long shape comparable to a comet or a torpedo. In this registration more than 80,000 heart beats are recorded. There is a white core in the point care diagram which represents normal and coherent heart rate variability. The bright blue coating and "clouds" around it indicate different stages of increased/decreased heart activity connected to exercises, emotional reactions and food intake.

Heart Rate Variability (HRV) Displays the Functional Heart's Intelligence

While the rhythmic beating of the heart was once believed to be monotonously regular, it was confirmed in 1968 that the rhythm of a healthy heart, even under resting conditions is surprisingly variable. This moment-to-moment, beat–to-beat variations between seemingly regular heartbeats are known as heart rate variability (HRV).

HRV is generated spontaneously by the healthy heart in response to changes in the breathing pattern, to the vibrations caused by the mechanical heartbeat and its propagation to the brain, changes in hormone levels, and changes in the activity of the immune system.

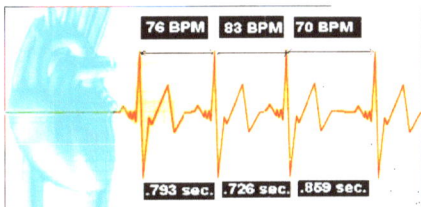

Figure 52 A section of an ECG reading with fundamental time measurements of heart rate variability HRV. It shows the small but countable differences between regular heartbeats.
Own work

The minimal time variations between heartbeats depend on the requirements for blood supply and oxygen utilization. The amount of blood which needs to be ejected relates to actual bodily and mental activity. Changing demand for blood supply modifies the length of muscular heart work and heart rate variability.

The small but relevant time differences between regular heartbeats can be easily overlooked when just the heart rate is measured and calculated. The HRV recording needs a special program recognizing small variations between the heartbeats within the ECG.

More specialized ECG programs contain the calculation of heart rate variability. It can be displayed as a pie diagram with three frequencies as it as displayed above.

HRV medical research has demonstrated measurable intelligence in the responses of the heart to changing conditions, and to the demanding impulses coming from within the body and from the environment. HRV is closely connected with the breathing mechanism, and with the brain's processing power. Your heart reacts according to the need for equilibrium in the autonomic nervous system, breathing capacity and the 24-hour circadian day and night cycle. HRV also reflects the intensity of hormonal activation and the activity of the immune system. It is well established that our physical and mental capabilities as well as level of physical health have a distinct impact on the HRV pattern.

Canadian scientist Dr Eugene Fischmann discovered heart rate variability, and published his findings in the American Heart Journal in 1968, Extensive further research evaluated many medical conditions and their relation to specific HRV patterns. HRV can be used for calculating the risk of sudden cardiac death (SCD).

HRV is extremely fine-tuned and has become a visual signature of the functioning of the intelligent heart. And importantly, this HRV data set can be obtained non-invasively, through the use of a standard 24 hours Holter ECG or through a short term registration lasting between 2 and 5 minutes.

Measuring HRV in real time is useful when monitoring complex physical training, and helps in evaluating the outcomes of such lifestyle modifications on the cardiovascular system. HRV is a measure of the individual's ability to cope with stress.

HF - is the frequency from 0.15 to 0.40 Hz
LF - is the frequency from 0.04 to 0.15 Hz
VLF- is the frequency below ⟨0.04 Hz

The **Hertz** (symbol Hz) is the unit of frequency in the international system of units (SI) and is defined as one cycle per second.

- The first of the measured HRV components is the high frequency (HF), which is coloured in deep blue. It mainly reflects lung function and the level of oxygenation of the body. This "sound of the lungs" can be heard using an acoustic instrument such as an stethoscope.
- The second HRV component is low frequency (LF). This "sound of the heart" relates to the heart function and it allows the estimation of the brain/heart cohesion and coordination. It can be heart only with a stethoscope.
- The third HRV component is an extremely gentle, inaudible "sound of endocrine and immune system". Even the release of hormones and bio-chemicals into blood stream can be recorded. It is displayed in green in the pie chart.

We are looking for a balanced distribution of the recorded frequencies. A balanced reading indicates healthy, normal functioning of the underlying physiological functions evaluated in this process of diagnostics. The ideal reading is where each frequency is roughly equal thirds and the chart takes on a shape similar to the well-known "Mercedes star" in the auto industry.

When the "Mercedes star" appears in the HRV record and the heart Cardio Image is close to the ideal pattern, it indicates a perfect moment for a woman to conceive and start a pregnancy. The heart Cardio Image is derived from hundreds of ECG registrations and colour mapped heart beats. HRV is displayed in colors as a "lead" of the Cardio Image and is generated as a Poincaré-Plot diagram. It is popularly known as a "comet" or a "torpedo".

An exact analysis of real time HRV registrations can reveal complex initial deviations in the cardiovascular system.

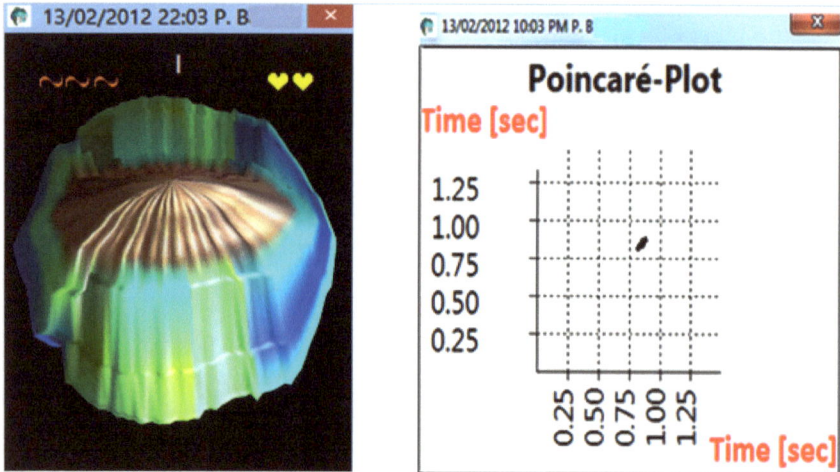

Figure 53 Cardio Image of a patient in a moment of stress as a brown at the core of the Cardio Image and and a limited HRV, a very small and short "torpedo/comet" indicated in the Poincaré-Plot diagram
Own work

The Cardio Image and limited HRV Poincaré-Plot diagram below were registered from a patient in a moment of a stress. He was suffering lower back pain and tightness in his chest. He could engaged only in minimal bodily exercise. His breathing pattern was very shallow and his breath was moving predominantly in the upper part of his chest. His mind could hardly focus and produced a high level of anxiety.

The scan shows a pattern of a strongly activated distressed pattern with the cardio stress index CSI elevated at 56%. (Acceptable values of the CSI are considered to be lower than 20%). The increased stress level shows as brown colour at the core of the heart Cardio Image, instead of blue-green.

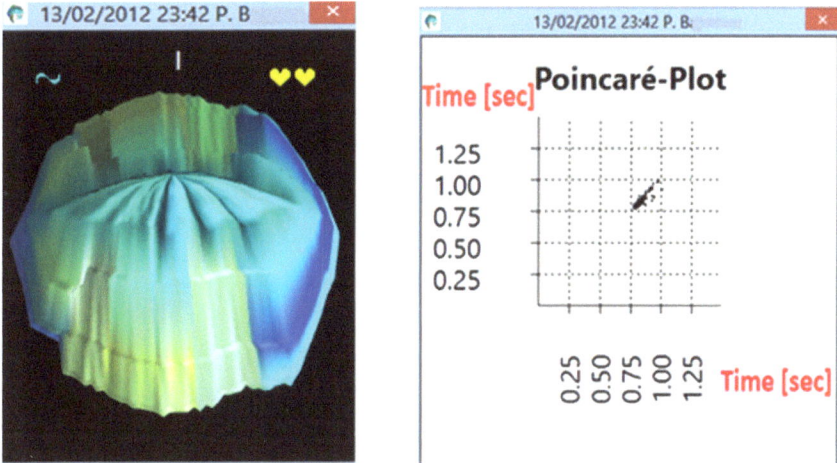

Figure 54 The Cardio Image displayed above originates from the same patient .After treatment with medical acupuncture and a short respiratory muscle training the patient's profile returned to normal indicated by the green color at the core of the Cardio Image and improved in the HRV Poincaré-Plot diagram indicated as a bigger and longer "torpedo/comet"

A follow up cardio check was recorded from the same patient after respiratory muscle training (RMT), medical acupuncture and a few minutes of rest.

Notice the relevant change in colours of the heart Cardio Image. Cardiovascular related distress has diminished. The reduction of cardio stress index (CSI) from 56% to 9 % brought the change in colours of the "lead" at the core of the Cardio Image. It turned from brown to blue and green. This shows a dramatic improvement in HRV, related heart's intelligence. It is valuable feedback to the patient and to the doctor/therapist.

On the right side is the Poincare Plot from the same test, the broader and longer the shape of the HRV "comet/torpedo", the better. A long comet/torpedo indicates optimal intelligent heart functionality. The elevated levels of circulating stress hormones have been inactivated and the stress cascade has stopped. The stress level reduction causes muscle relaxation, the return of harmonious diaphragmatic breathing and a full normalization of the oxygen supply.

The human heart's intelligence has been evident for centuries but now it can be measured and displayed using 21st century technology.

The Intelligent Pattern of Heart Rate Variability

A high performing body produces a stronger heartbeat and more blood volume is ejected throughout the system. A less active body results in a weaker and shorter lasting period between two heartbeats, ejecting less blood volume.

No two heartbeats are the same. Every heartbeat has different characteristics in time. It expresses the actual strength of the heart muscle and is the individual's signature in action. The HRV Poincaré-Plot is a useful view of the heart's intelligence, manifesting cumulative life experience, age, gender and the cardiovascular regulation patterns written in the individual DNA.

Limitations of the Heart's Intelligence

Measuring heart rate variability (HRV) creates a dynamic window in real time to observe the heart's interactions with the brain, the independent, autonomic nervous system, breathing activity and biochemical-hormone stimulation. HRV is also an important indicator for resilience in training and behavioural flexibility. It reflects the individual's capability to adapt effectively to stress and to challenging environmental impacts.

Many research studies have examined HRV patterns in a wide range of dysfunctional conditions. Altered and limited HRV has been associated with a range of medical conditions including:

- Hypertension (Schroedere.B, Liao, Chambless, Prineas, Evans, & Heiss, 2003)
- Arrhythmias (Task force of the European Society of Cardiology and the North American Society of Pacing and Electrophysiology, 1996)
- Autoimmune disorders (Ljudmila, 2009)
- Environmental sensitivity (Park, et al., 2007)
- Chronic pain (Adeyemi EOA, 1999)
- Fibromyalgia (Mehmet Tolga Doğru, 2009)
- Chronic fatigue (Kohichi Takamoto1, 2009)
- Anxiety disorders (Licht Carmilla M. M., 2009)
- Clinical depression (Freedland, 2009)
- Post-traumatic stress disorders (Kearya Therese A, 2009)
- Sleep related breathing disorders (Sields Robert W, 2009)
- Breathing techniques (Chalayea P., 2009) (Del Pozo Jessica M., 2004)
- Disturbances of autonomic regulation and orthostatic deregulation by astronauts after short duration space flights (Blaber Andrew P, 2004)
- Heart Rate Variability and adult personality: A nationally representative study ((Čukić I, April 2014)
- Genetics and HRV, the COMT gene polymorphism in Depression (Woody, McGeary, & Gibb, 2014)
- Genome and HRV in relation to Sudden Cardiac Death (Ilkka Seppälä, 2013)
- Panic attacks, genotype and HRV and (Agorastos Agorastosa, 2014)
- Brain Derived Neurotropic Factor (gene and HVR (Marosi K, 2013)
- New Cardio Stress Theory (Dyczynski J. Sleptsova-Freidrich I., Rudhart –Dyczynski Angela published in 2010, 2011 and 2014)

An limited HRV pattern is also often found in the normal aging process of humans. The study published in 1999 by Sirkku Pikkujämsä from the University Hospital of Oulu in Finland entitled "Heart Rate Variability and Baroreflex Sensitivity in Subjects without Heart Diseases", examines the effects of age, sex and cardiovascular risk factors on the HRV patterns. Dr Pikkujämsä found large inter-individual variations of HRV patterns from childhood to middle age. In the course of aging the diversity and the strength of HRV components are in decline. The most reduced components of HRV during the aging process are related to breathing and lung function (low frequency LF component) and the heart/brain related (the high frequency HF) component.

Acupuncture and Respiratory Muscle Training (RMT) Can Normalize Abnormal HRV

The human body produces a stress hormones such as adrenaline or noradrenaline on and off throughout a normal day. But adrenal overstimulation can make the heart rhythm more rigid and it can even induce a spasm of a coronary artery. This can result in HRV can decreasing, even to a point where it is unreadable.

An excess of stress hormones can also reduce the amount of blood that is actually being pumped through the heart. The amount of blood that is pumped by each heartbeat is measured as "the ejection fraction", or EF. EF is a measurement, expressed as a percentage, of how much blood the left ventricle pumps out with each contraction. An ejection fraction of 55 % means that from the all blood filling the left chamber 55 percent is pushed out with each heartbeat.

Consider now the case of Steve, a patient who presented with chest symptoms, anxiety and disturbed sleep. During examination Steve exhibited superficial breathing and complained about burning in the chest and heaviness. Steve had been exposed to professional stress as a teacher.

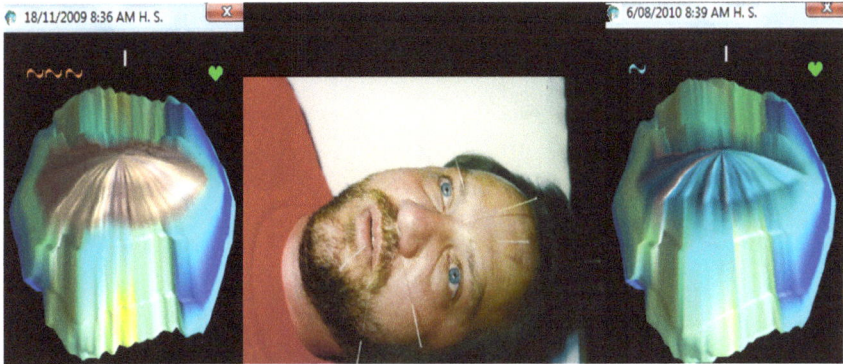

55 Heart Cardio Images of a patient before and after treatment. The Cardio Image on the left reflects a stressful situation. Increased stress is displayed as the brown coloration at the core, the "lead" of the heart Cardio Image on the left side. The Cardio Image on the right was recorded after respiratory muscle training (RMT) and medical acupuncture, about 1 hour later. The green/blue colour of the follow up Cardio Image registration indicated the return of patient's normal profile
Own work

The heart Cardio Image on the left reflects a stressful situation of the patient. The cardio stress index (CSI) was measured at 70%, which is far above the acceptable values of 20 % or less. Increased stress is displayed as the brown coloration at the core, the "lead" of the heart portrait image. The cardio portrait image on the right was recorded after respiratory muscle training (RMT) and medical acupuncture, about 1 hour later. The relevant changes in colour confirm the normalization of the blood supply and a reduction of CSI from 70% to 12%.

By utilising the Cardio Images Steve was able to see a visual representation of the changing condition of his heart – before and after treatment. This feedback helped him to maintain the positive change. Steve had more colour in his cheeks and, directly after the intervention, he felt more energetic, yet calm and peaceful.

ECG: Electrocardiogram (ECG)

Since the scientific discovery of the ECG in 1901, the recordings of the heart electrical activity, the excitation of the heart's muscle became the most common and valuable diagnostic technique in cardiology performed millions times a day around the world. The electromagnetic function of the heart is a constant function necessary for every activity of the human life.

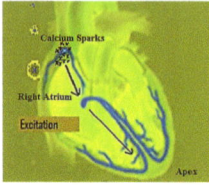

Figure 56 Electrical impulses in the heart are caused by Calcium sparks initiating every heart beat
Own work

Electrical impulses are caused by calcium sparks initiating every single heartbeat. It ignites a flow of current in the upper heart chamber, called right atrium. Then the electrical impulse travels downward alongside the blue marked pathways to the Apex, the tip of the heart.

The ECG reading is a precise and an irreplaceable diagnostic technique to assess heart function. ECG recordings are currently used in all clinical investigations of heart disorders. An ECG is always done when the integrity of the heart and cardiovascular risks need to be assessed.

Angina pectoris is a symptom of coronary artery blockage, sometimes described as a tightness of the chest or heart palpitations. It produces typical changes in the ECG curve. The early recognition of heart attack trough ECG is recommended in all guidelines of national and international cardiac societies as the first step in cardiovascular diagnostics.

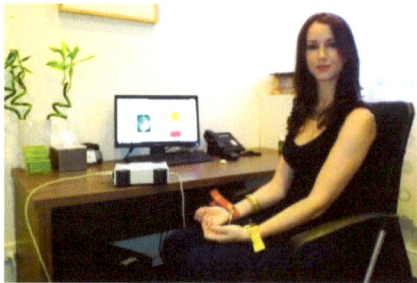

Figure 57 Registration of Cardio Image and HRV using Vicardio
Own work

An ECG device measures the gentle biological current generated by the heart muscle and indicates its electromagnetic vector, or direction. The electrical potentials from the heart travel down to the hands and legs. The ECG leads collect the impulses from the ankles and wrists to be converted and amplified in the ECG device into a specific reading.

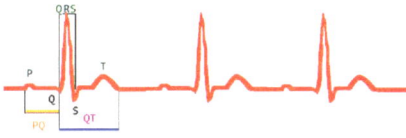

Figure 58 A typical healthy pattern of an ECG reading. It shows four waves originating from the initial excitation, mechanical contraction and relaxation of the heart muscle

P-wave reflects the initial excitation of the pre-chambers and the contraction of two heart's atria pumping the blood flow downwards to the heart chambers.

Q-wave is a negative deflection that precedes the R spike and represents electrical activation of the interventricular septum separating the left and right chamber of the heart.

QRS-spike is an expression of the excitation and contraction of both heart chambers, reflecting the time of blood flow ejection from the chambers into the aorta, the biggest blood vessel outgoing from the heart, which supplies the whole body with fresh blood and oxygen

T-wave is the electrical manifestation of the relaxation of the heart. At this time the relaxed heart is re-filled with new oxygenated blood from the lungs

The normal record of the ECG will show the perfect timing and the highest precision of the heart. The human heart is able to coordinate electrical and mechanical functions. It works 24/7 without any break. The heart processes incoming big data, relevant for the functioning of the body and surrounding environment and its intelligence calculates in a fraction of a second all the necessary parameters to supply the entire body, all vital internal organs, with an adequate amount of blood, energy and oxygen.

One Complete Cycle of Heart's Electrical Activity: Excitation, Contraction and Relaxation

One complete cycle of the heart's electrical activity has three phases known as electrical **excitation**, mechanical **contraction** and **relaxation**.

Excitation involves the spontaneous generation of the electrical impulse and its propagation throughout the entire heart muscle the electromagnetic excitation starts with calcium sparks. The initial impulse is generated under the influence of light, bio-photons, and chemical and electromagnetic forces in the left atrium (left pre-chamber). The spontaneous electrical excitation spreads down alongside a muscular septum which separates the left and right chambers of the heart, and this propagating electrical impulse causes the heart muscle to contract. The spontaneous, regular heart rhythm is generated at the basal rate of 50 to 60 heartbeats a minute in a resting position. Depending on the body's activity, the heart rhythm can accelerate to 150 or 180 beats in a minute during a high level of physical training.

Every electrical excitation is followed by a mechanical contraction. The left chamber ejects about 50 ml of oxygenated blood into the circulation. The mechanical force of the heartbeat generates the pulse and pressure wave. The oxygen in fresh blood is utilized immediately in the tissues in the process of cellular breathing. Fresh blood also carries the supply of minerals and nutrients. At the same time the identical amount of utilized blood is ejected from the right heart chamber into the lungs for the process of re-oxygenation.

In the mechanical relaxation phase the heart is filled with oxygenated blood from the lungs.

A complete cycle of the heart's activity (electrical excitation, mechanical contraction and relaxation) can be registered as an **ECG complex**.

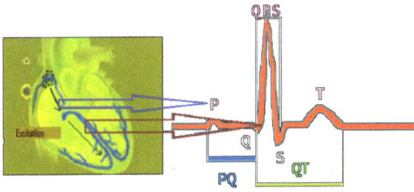

Figure 59 Diagram shows a complete ECG complex and the origin of the P wave- contraction of the atria, ORS complex-contraction of the chambers and the T wave-relaxation of the heart chambers

The ECG complex includes the P-wave relating to the activity of the pre-chambers (atria), the QRS-spike reflecting the contraction of the heart muscle and the T-wave occurring during the mechanical relaxation of the heart. The time related to the contraction and relaxation of the heart's chambers is called a QT time. It is counted from the beginning of the negative deflection known as the Q wave and it finishes at the end of the T wave. This time can be affected by many drugs and supplements in a negative way causing the long QT syndrome causing the delay in the mechanical relaxation of the heart. Long QT syndrome is one of the risk factors for the sudden cardiac death SCD.

The core diagnostic tools are:

1. ECG,
2. Cardio Image,
3. heart rate variability HRV, and
4. blood pressure

But the level of oxygen saturation of the blood is also important in monitoring of the efficiency of your breathing technique.

Oxygen Saturation

Pulse oximetry is a non-invasive method to monitor blood oxygen saturation. Importantly, rather than just getting a "snapshot" reading, you can wear a pulse oximeter while training to keep an eye on your oxygen saturation in real time. At the same time the pulse oximeter shows your pulse rate. It is an ideal device to monitor the progress of your daily respiratory muscle training.

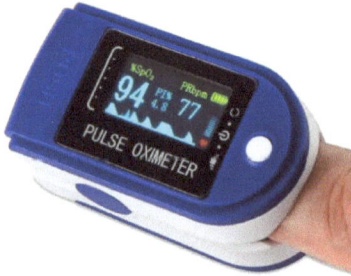

After the finger is placed into the device you need a couple of minutes to get a stable average reading. Your target blood oxygen saturation during RMT is between 98 and 99%.

Figure 60 Image of a finger pulse oximeter. The bigger number 94 indicates the oxy-gen blood saturation and 77 is the pulse rate
Obn work

MRI Scans

You should learn more about curative magnetics by delving into evidenced-based conventional and non-conventional scientific sources.

Modern medical diagnostics can collect near perfect MRI images of our heart, which are very useful for diagnostics. It helps the individual imagination to zoom down to the structural organ level.

The contemporary operating magnetic resonance imaging (MRI) machines develop a magnetic strength of 1 to 3 or even 7 Tesla. An MRI machine with the strength of 2 Tesla produces a magnetic field which is 30,000 times stronger than the magnetic field of the Earth. The MRI machine, which is generating 3 Tesla electromagnetic field is 60,000 times stronger than the electromagnetic field of our entire earth. More than 36,000 MRI machines worldwide are in operation, and in the USA alone, in 2019 over 40 million MRI scans, in Germany 12 million, in Japan 10 million, in France 9 million, UK 4 million were performed. Worldwide in 2019 more than 100 million MRI scans were ordered by physicians and performed by radiologists. More details about the diagnostic and curative value of MRI will be discussed in following chapter.

Book 2: The Quantum Heart

1. *Medical Physics*

According to the Australasian College of Physical Scientist & Engineers in Medicine Medical Physics is a branch of applied physics which employs physical concepts for the prevention, diagnosis and treatment of human disease. It is a truly diverse field that utilises the knowledge gained in other areas of physics and applies it to heal people.

https://www.acpsem.org.au/Meet-Our-Members/Medical-Physics

A new Understanding of Healing

Quantum physics deals with the behaviour of the universe at the smallest scale. While classical physics successfully describes and explains the behaviour of larger things like rocks, water, wind, people, planets and galaxies, it is hard pressed to account for what happens at the atomic and subatomic level. Down there, things behave strangely, but they work to utmost perfection.

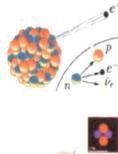

Figure 61 The quantum probability approach is at least as important in medicine and in our daily lives as the four forces of nature set out in fundamental physics: electromagnetic field, gravitation, weak interaction between particles and atomic strong interaction
Own work

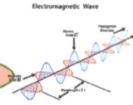

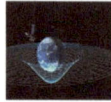

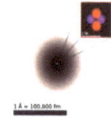

The principles of quantum physics were first articulated more than 120 years ago, and now quantum physics is a defining cornerstone of 21st century science. The electromagnetic field uncovered by medical physics has been used broadly for more than 80 years and it is one of the four fundamental forces of the universe.

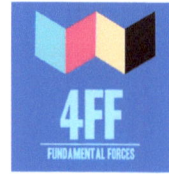

Contemporary science has greatly expanded our understanding of the human heart. Recent discoveries have taken knowledge beyond the intelligent heart, and even the ancient traditional Chinese medicine concept of *shen* is translated as "Spirit" or "Mind." The *shen* is responsible for consciousness, cognition, emotional life and our "presence". Chinese medicine emphasises the importance of addressing both the physical and mental/spiritual aspects of disease, addressing the spiritual aspects of the heart.

Medical physics opens our sensibility to the quantum world and the hidden realm of the vast universe which is inaccessible to our senses. It transformed our physical world and created an extended reality by the means of smart phones, computers health oriented electronic devices. Quantum physics is the science of light. (A quantum is the smallest amount of light emitted by an energized particle known as electron). Quantum reality has different laws, which are not in agreement with the laws of conventional physics that we experience in 3D space-time. The enigmatic fabric of the Universe is an invisible dimension of subatomic particles and probability waves. It is a world of unlimited potentiality in creation of health and wealth. Quantum physics has led to astounding advances in engineering, physics and medicine in the past 20 years. Devices such as medical lasers, mobile phones, apps for cardio monitoring, watches tracking our bio-functions, superconductors and GPS technology all exploit the laws of quantum physics. The principles of quantum physics have been applied in medicine, photochemistry, high-resolution microscopy, optical imaging and optical communication, nano-medication, and in the measurement of molecular distances. Recently, entangled particles and photons have been used to build silicon crystal-based supercomputers, robotics, artificial intelligence, and extremely sharp imaging techniques in medicine. Google and the central intelligence agency (CIA) operate their quantum computers since 2011 Sometime this century we will have a general-purpose quantum computer for everybody which will be able to perform its operations at un unprecedented super high-speed.

The probabilistic approach and unusual behaviour of subatomic particles energized by photons of light do not fit into the map of the three-dimensional world and the 3D space-time used by our conditioned minds. "Like powerful sorcerers, all humans can see the future—not a clear and determined future, but a murky, probabilistic one" (Jonathan Gottschall).

One of the most advanced visual art displaying the 3D space-time governed by the conditioned mind and the underlying unlimited life giving force, the fabric of the Universe accessible by the heart and spirit is the film "Matrix". The story incorporates references to numerous philosophical, religious, or spiritual ideas, among others the dilemma of choice vs. control, the brain in a vat thought experiment, messianism, and the concepts of inter-dependency and love. The films focus on the plight of Neo (Keanu Reeves), Trinity (Carrie-Anne Moss), and Morpheus (Laurence Fishburne) trying to free humanity from the system while pursued by its guardians of artificial intelligence (AI). https://en.wikipedia.org/wiki/The_Matrix_(franchise)

Medical physics in its application to healthcare for body imaging like the magnetic resonance imaging (MRI) can create such precise and detailed pictures of the body interior never seen before. Even the function of the heart and brain and their processing power became visible. The quantum related measurements and their application for new sophisticated treatments revolutionized medical approaches to diagnostics and changed the medical curative landscape. It determines now how we treat illness in the 21st century.

The new discipline of medical physics is studying the superconductive abilities of the human body. This property of a material occurs in some materials when they lose their resistance. Under special circumstances elements such as silicon or boron behave not more like electrical wire during a flow of an electric current, they act as a superconducting computer chip. It means that for example the impulses in the human body can be conducted instantly without barriers and at high speed.

We are interacting with the Universe and we are a dynamic part of it.

Medical physics aims to better understand the process activation of the superconductive bio-substances contained in the human body such as silicon or the less predictable boron in the process known as doping. This is an example how medical physics addresses the unlimited probability approach in treatments of conditions which could be classified as quantum illness.

The heart acts as the master connection between 3D oriented space-time and the hidden electromagnetic dimension the fabric of the Universe.

Recent ground-breaking discoveries in quantum physics, medical physics and in cardiology align with ancient traditional Chinese medicine ("TCM"), which considers the human heart to be the emperor of our body and the storehouse of the spirit.

The TCM yin and yang view of the universe has much in common with relativity theory and quantum physics. TCM teaches us that the universe is in ultimate balance with the human body. The human body is yin and it is linked with Earth, the ultimate yin in the Chinese characterisation of the universe. The spirit, *shen*, residing in the heart, belongs to the category yang, and it can access heaven, which is the ultimate yang. Both yin and yang are in a relative balance which determines perfect health.

The body and the spirit connect at conception and birth, and they separate in the process of death. Intuitively we know that we are connected to the fabric of the Universe. We interact with the Universe and we are a dynamic part of it. Sometimes we shape it. Sometimes we have a special feeling of all-inclusiveness. This state of bliss has been experienced by many allied health practitioners, qi-gong instructors and the famous yogis practicing regular training and meditation. But also by anyone who fell in love. Such a time of universal integrity of the body, soul, mind, heart and spirit constitutes perfect consciousness. This holistic perfection can also be experienced during a medical acupuncture treatment, during deep meditation or during intense prayer.

Heart science is expanding beyond Cardiology and the mechanical functionality of the heart. A new medical field of neurocardiology is emerging, which studies the connections between heart and brain. Harvard's Dr John Hagelin is a leading quantum physicist who has revealed the connection between universal consciousness and the fabric of the Universe in his well-known public presentations.

2. Quantum Heart and Body

The human heart is much more than a precise mechanical system pumping the blood and supplying the body with oxygen and nutrients. The human heart communicates with the dimensions of physics known as an electromagnetic field and with of the fabric of the Universe revealed by quantum physics. The fabric of the Universe is connected to the genuine reality of very small spaces and unimaginable small fractions of time, as it is defined in modern quantum physics.

The metaphysical aspects of heart encompass its ability to operate in the invisible field of consciousness. The spirit is the tool which is designed to explore and to develop the field of the individual consciousness. This is the probability approach in the modern life of 21st century and the quantum world of unlimited potentiality in the fabric of the Universe for health.

Every divine encounter with the fabric of the Universe is made and conducted by the intelligence of the human heart. The heart cooperates intensely with the invisible unified field of bio-photons, subatomic particles, and electromagnetic waves.

3. Timeline and Discovery of Quantum Physics

Quantum Leaping Electrons

The electron is the most intriguing particle in the Universe. It constitutes electricity and electric power. Electricity is a form of energy resulting from the existence of moving electron particles. The dynamically flowing stream of electrons is known as an electric current. Electricity is the backbone of modern industrial society. It exhibits extraordinary versatility and has almost limitless applications which include transport, heating, lighting, communications and computation.

The electron was discovered 124 years ago, not long before the emergence of quantum physics. The decoding of the electron's enigmatic behaviour let to the development of the new discipline known as quantum physics. The new rules applying to quantum reality and to the probability approach enabled scientists and doctors to better understand the invisible world of the fabric of the Universe. Now the achievements of medical physics are used in modern medical diagnostics and treatment. The superposition of an energized electron and the twin concept of quantum entanglement within unlimited potentiality modified our perception of healing and the functioning of the human body. The human heart and the human body function according to these quantum reality laws.

In 1896, the British physicist J. J. Thomson, with his colleagues John S. Townsend and H. A. Wilson discovered that an electrically charged piece of metal in a hollow lamp emits mobile particles. Up to that moment, it was believed that radiant energy was made up of waves or atoms, but this simple experiment changed everything.

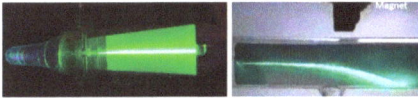

Figure 62 **The path of the electron beam is curved in a magnetic field**
Cathode Ray Tube by Pseudo1ntellectual
https://www.youtube.com/
watch?v=7YHwMWcxeX8

It could be debated that these pioneering physicists were in fact the first quantum physicists. They produced a stream of charged electrons forming a jet of energy and emitting visible light. Furthermore, this jet of energy and light could be influenced and redirected by a simple magnet.

This discovery was followed by extensive research into this radiant energy and the Nobel Prize in physics in 1918 was awarded to German physicist Max Planck, "in recognition of the services he rendered to the advancement of physics by his discovery of energy quanta." The word "quanta" is the plural from of "quantum", hence the term "quantum physics."

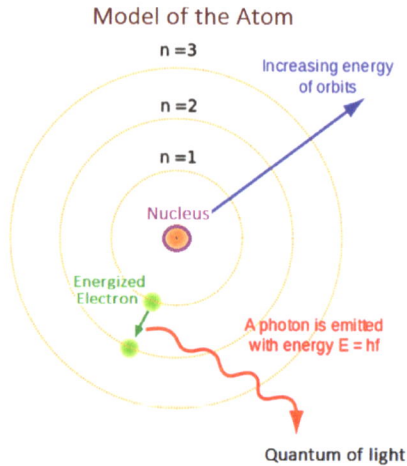

Figure 63 Niels Bohr's quantum model
of an atom with electrons changing their
orbits and emitting quanta of light
modified
Wiki Commons by JabberWok

Planck was one of the most important physicists of the 20th Century. In 1900 he discovered that light and other electromagnetic waves were emitted in an exceedingly small packet of energy that he called quantum. And a quantum is the tiniest bit of light absorbed by an energized electron. When an electron emits a quantum of energy in form of a photon it means that it returns to normal state from the energized superposition.

This discovery inspired Professor Niels Bohr to develop a quantum model of the atom rewarded in 1922 with the Nobel Prize in physics. His achievement highlighted the existence of quantum reality and the prize was an acknowledgement of quantum physics by the global scientific community.

Superposition

In Niels Bohr's atom model the electrons are moving around the core of the atom, the nucleus. An electron absorbing the smallest quantum of energy, a photon, becomes an energized electron and it moves from its normal position to a higher energy state inheriting more energy known as the superposition. This is the basis of cellular respiration where energised electrons make energy https://en.wikipedia.org/wiki/Electron_transport_chain

Quantum Leap

The superposition allows the particle to carry information and to build unlimited connections to other particles. From the superposition the energized electron can enter 3D space-time and is not limited in space. The energized electron does not move in one direction, as you would expect. Instead the energized electron can make an unpredictable jump from one place to another, and this kind of jump is called a quantum leap.

So, an energized electron can appear anywhere in the human body. It can overcome any biological barriers like cell membranes or fascia. It can also jump to any place in the Universe. This feature of the energized electron constitutes the unlimited potentiality in healing.

The quantum leap quickly became famous and controversial as it was at odds with established classical physics. It just made no sense to classical physicists that a particle could vanish from one location and simultaneously appear somewhere else without it having traversed the space between the two locations. The most astonishing thing for physicists was, and is, the fact that an energized and accelerated electron disappears and literally becomes for a moment a virtual particle, utterly undetectable.

So, what really happens during the quantum leap? And how it can be interpreted?

Black Holes

Without the probability approach we will never understand this mystery in physics. It seems to be that the energized electron leaps into the invisible 5th electromagnetic dimension. The 5th dimension is hidden because it is placed beside or outside of our tangible 3D space-time. These hidden realms have been known for about a century; however the term "black hole" was coined by the physicist John Wheeler at a conference on nuclear physics in 1967

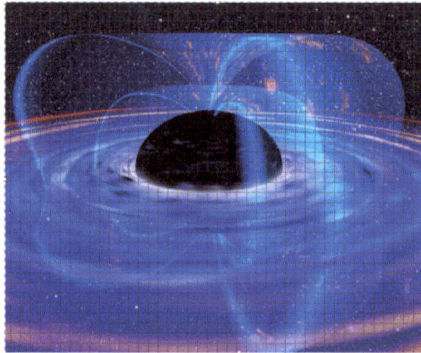

Figure 64 Artist's impression of a black hole system
Image Credit: Dana Berry, NASA

Quantum leap of the energized electron into black holes

"The quantum leap of the energized electron into black holes" is an intuitive explanation, which I developed in 2015. This hypothesis was discussed at the Gravity Discovery Centre in Gingin, Western Australia at the 9th Australasian Conference on General Relativity and Gravitation, 27 to 30 November 2017 It theorises that, in the moment of energy absorption, an energized electron enters the hidden, electromagnetic dimension, reaching its superposition. It may be that it enters one of the black holes existing alongside 3D space-time. Black holes are invisible. Space telescopes with the most sophisticated special lenses observing the cosmos from space cannot see black holes. The ultra-modern Hubble telescope can help to identify and locate black holes based on the configuration of those bodies located close to black holes. Astronomers can only infer the presence of a black hole in each location because of the odd behaviour and positioning of the surrounding stars.

Professor Leonard Susskind, a renowned expert on black holes and quantum field theory, states that information is indestructible and that all the information we create gathers in black holes, where it is stored and is not accessible now.

The Fabric of the Universe

One energized electron is a tiny part of the massive movement of the trillions of electrons that make a quantum leap in the smallest moment in time. We cannot imagine the amount of energy created by these energized electron waves. These uncountable numbers of electron quantum leaps creating movements like a wave form the fabric of the Universe with its unlimited potentiality.

Multitudes of electrons dwell in the hidden electromagnetic dimension outside of 3D space-time in a state of superposition and wait for a signal to re-enter 3D space-time, to materialize anywhere into the 3D reality, including the human body and the heart. In the human body electrons are not flowing along a wire; instead, an electrical charge jumps from one cell to the next until it reaches its destination. The ultimate jumper for the heart is located in the right atrium, and it controls the rhythm of heartbeat and the movement of blood from the heart to every other part of the body according to the study performed by Fish R.M at al. Energized electrons travel in space-time, and are not bound to a specific location. They are hidden from researchers whose equipment is limited to operating only in 3D space-time. The fact that an energized electron cannot be tracked down by existing technology in our well known 3D space-time lends support to the theory that quantum leap of the energized electron crosses from the 3D space-time into the invisible electromagnetic dimension of the fabric of the Universe.

Probability Waves

Probability waves are the foundation of quantum reality and they create the unlimited potential for health addressed by medical physics.

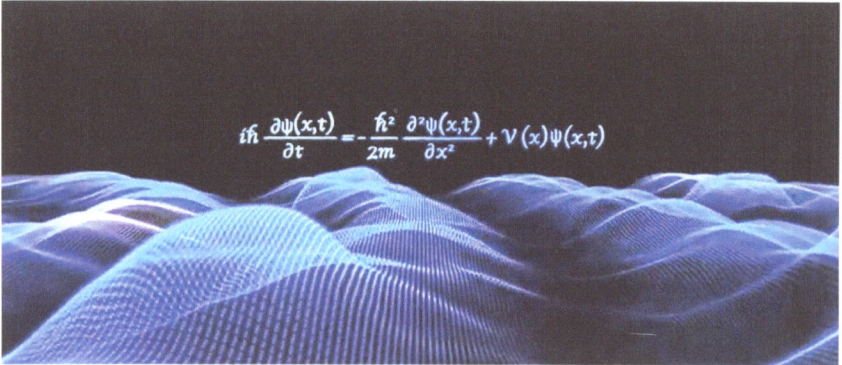

$$i\hbar \frac{\partial \psi(x,t)}{\partial t} = -\frac{\hbar^2}{2m}\frac{\partial^2 \psi(x,t)}{\partial x^2} + V(x)\psi(x,t)$$

65. Probability waves of the fabric of the Universe and the equation describing it
This image is credited to video quantum world and reality, World Science Festival. https://www.youtube.com/watch?v=GdqC2bVLesQ.

It is an exciting prospect for medical science to explore and use the quantum probability approach to medicine.

4. *The Revolutionary ASPECT Experiment in Paris*

The controversy between the views of Nils Bohr and Albert Einstein concerning the role of the Quantum Observer needed more than 60 years to be clarified. The dogma that the speed of light is the highest speed existing in our universe, as stated by Einstein, has been increasingly questioned by physicists and quantum scientists. Subsequent research has confirmed the existence of informational entanglement with the exchange of information at a speed faster than light.

The French physicist Alain Aspect performed a famous experiment in 1982 known as the ASPECT experiment.[https://www.oxfordreference.com/view/10.1093/oi/authority.20110803095429178

It has changed irreversibly the perception of quantum reality and confirmed the existence of the fabric of the Universe. The ASPECT experiment proved the quantum nature of the reality. It confirmed that nothing in the universe—solid particles such as photons and electrons, atoms nor the universe itself—has a definite form until are measured.

The ASPECT's outcomes challenge us to redefine our role as humans in the world of 3D space-time in which we live. It teaches us the importance of the spiritual part of life beyond 3D reality. We govern our own health and reign on planet Earth according to our intensions aligned with the laws of medical physics.

It turns out that humans are more powerful than we ever thought. We can shape our bodily 3D space-time reality and we have the capacity to receive and exchange information from the quantum reality of the fabric of the Universe. We can transform it to intelligent information through our quantum heart and we can develop a superior mind.

By careful analysis of the results of the ASPECT study the scientists performing and observing the experiments became aware that they make a dynamic contribution to their results simply by virtue of being present and observing. The observer of an experiment is not neutral. The observer has a big, measurable impact on the outcome of a study, based on their intentional interactions with the fabric of the Universe. The outcomes of ASPECT stimulated fundamental discussions about:

- The impact of the engaged researcher as a Quantum Observer in medical studies
- Real intention as an important tool in medical trials
- The dominant intentional frequency in the study can produce a desired outcome

Medical experiments usually involve many observers: the funding organizations, pharmaceutical companies, universities, and the scientists allied with pharmaceutical multinationals. Contemporary, multi-centre studies might include thousands of patients, and many teams of researchers. Most medical studies begin with the intention to prove the effectiveness of a certain medication or to predict an intended outcome after a specific medical intervention.

Prior to performing an experiment, scientists must model the experiment as a conceptual construct. The managers have to consider it for a viable and profitable business model. Based on the calculations the managers must project the revenue and estimate the financial risks and potential profits. The desired outcome of the study is projected as information into the fabric of the Universe and will move the energy pattern in the quantum reality in the desired direction. Therefore the outcomes of medical studies confirm this universal law of medical physics:

"Observation with directed intention results in a specific manifestation."

5. The Electromagnetic Model of the Universe

Superstrings

For almost 100 years quantum physics has been exploring the 5th, hidden electromagnetic dimension, the fabric of the Universe. The discovery made by Dr Kaluza confirmed that the fundamental forces of nature can be unified. His concept of a 5th, electromagnetic dimension became the foundation of the modern superstrings model of the fabric of the Universe.

This 5th dimension exists beside our 3D space-time reality. The superstrings theory unifies the fundamental forces of nature into one electromagnetic field. It also predicts the existence of many invisible dimensions.

In a nutshell, the superstring theory sees the fabric of the Universe built from unimaginably small, vibrating superstrings. The theory reveals the enormous plasticity and dynamics of our vast universe.

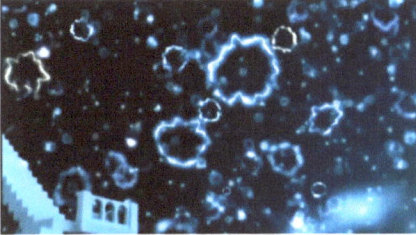

Figure 66 Superstrings of the fabric of the Universe.
. This image is credited to video quantum world and reality, World Science Festival. https://www.youtube.com/ watch?v=GdqC2bVLesQ

Based on this new model we can see how the fabric of the Universe can be activated by an intention, operating at an ultra-high speed beyond our imagination. Superstrings resonate with our directed intentions and specific intentional observations. This process is ongoing, building up and collapsing in trillions of probability waves in a friction of a second in the fabric of the Universe. In his 2011 bestseller, *The Hidden Reality*, Brian Green says:

Permeating the universe is a magnetic field, thousands of times stronger than that created in our most advanced MRI machines, and one that cannot be switched off by a technician.

Dr Greene's superstrings theory is literally shifting the stars and the universe.

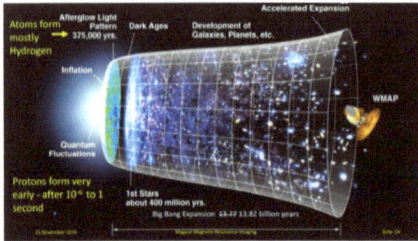

Figure 67 Timeline of the universe. In this diagram, time passes from left to right, so at any given time, the universe is represented by a disk-shaped "slice" of the diagram

Wiki Commons NASA,Science Team - Original version: NASA; modified by Cherkash, Public Domain

Other physicists performed intense research on the electromagnetic nature of the universe and found that our universe is expanding. In other words, "It had been it is, and it will be." Three scientists shared in 2011 the Nobel Prize for physics for this scientific work: Dr Saul Perlmutter, Dr Adam Riess and Dr Brian Paul Schmidt.

The picture shows the expansion of electromagnetic energy within the Universe. The confirmation of the electromagnetic universe was made through observations of distant stars called supernovae. A supernova is a huge astronomical event that occurs during the last stage of a star's life. A supernova collapses in a final titanic explosion and releases a staggering amount of electromagnetic energy. This causes the sudden appearance of a "new bright star" we can experience in our lifetime.

Modern medicine has been using strong electromagnetic fields in diagnostics for more than 35 years. Magnetic resonance imaging (MRI) is used to visualize the whole human body and its internal organs. The MRI applies boron-based magnets, but how does MRI work? How it is possible to visualize the human body by applying an external electromagnetic field? Dr Richard Ansorge from the Cavendish Laboratory at Cambridge University explains it in his power point presentations. http://people.bss.phy.cam.ac.uk/~rea1/

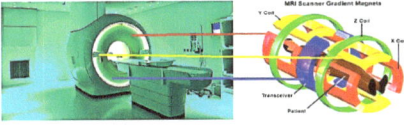

Figure 68 Modern MRI scanner and the MRI scanner gradient magnets
Image credited to Amber Diagnostics

An MRI scanner works on small mini-magnets that occur naturally in the water of every cell of the human body. The nano-magnet at the atomic level is a positive charged proton, the core of the of the hydrogen atom. The hydrogen atom is the simplest of all atoms. It is the first in the periodic table of elements and has the symbol H. It is most common element of our universe, a part of a water molecule. About 75% of all the matter in the universe is built from hydrogen. Most of the organic molecules, e.g. fat, sugars and proteins are also rich in hydrogen atoms. Water (H_2O) contains two hydrogen and one oxygen atom and constitutes 70% of the mass of human body. Hydrogen protons are the fundamental particles of the human body. One atom of hydrogen consists of one positively charged proton (+) and one negative electron (-). The proton sits in the centre of the atom and is spinning constantly, producing electrical charge and an accompanying magnetic field.

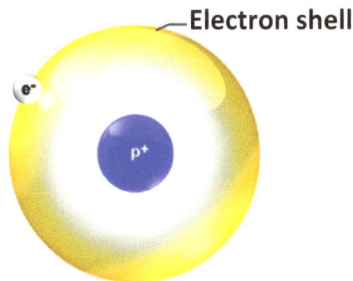

Hydrogen - 1
mass number :1

69 Hydrogen atom
Wiki Commons by Bruce Blaus Blausen

The orbiting, negative charged electron is in a perfect balance with the Hydrogen proton, the core of the atom. Even in the core in the atom are the electromagnetic forces connected to quarks. Quarks have a number of interesting properties, including electric charge, mass, colour charge, and spin. A proton is composed of two up quarks, one down quark, and the gluons that mediate the electromagnetic forces "binding" them together.

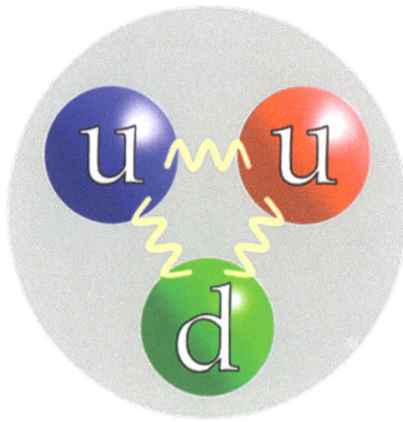

Figure 70 The quark structure of the proton
Wiki Commons by Arpad Horvath

1 ml of water contains more than 6 trilliards of protons, a number that is hard to imagine:

6,000,000,000,000,000,000,000. There are about 42 litres of water in an average human body weighing 70 kg, equivalent to 42,000 millilitres. Multiplication of that number by the amount of protons in one ml of water (that big number above), results in an unutterably large number of protons in each of us: It is 252,000,000,000,000,000,000,000,000. I don't even know how to say that number, but that's how many tiny magnets with a magnetic spin there are in the human body. All these nano-magnets have a random orientation. It is a part of a natural disorder in the world known as entropy.

During an MRI scan, all random directed nano-magnets in the body's water are aligned in one direction. The latest 2 Tesla MRI machine creates an electromagnetic field which is 60,000 stronger than the magnetic field of the Earth.

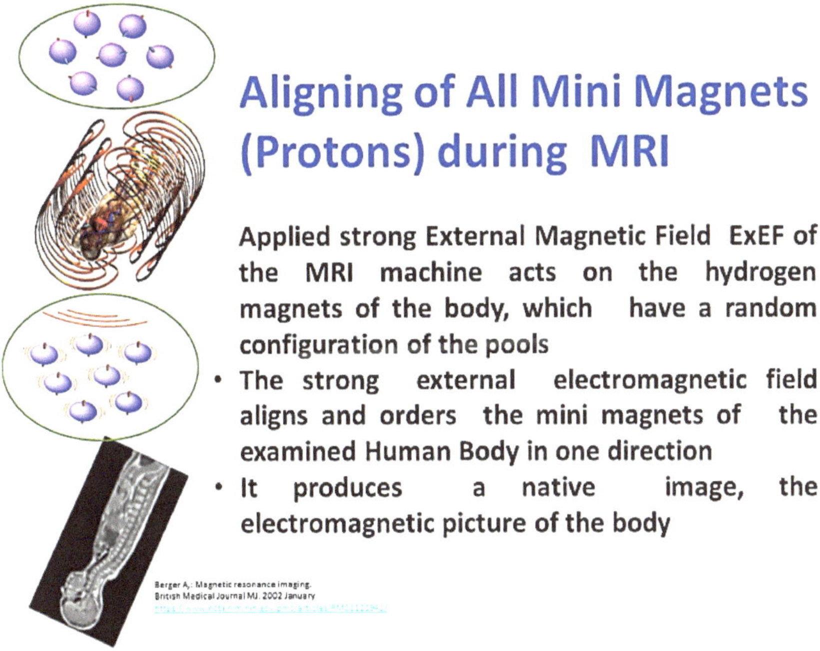

Aligning of All Mini Magnets (Protons) during MRI

Applied strong External Magnetic Field ExEF of the MRI machine acts on the hydrogen magnets of the body, which have a random configuration of the pools

- **The strong external electromagnetic field aligns and orders the mini magnets of the examined Human Body in one direction**
- **It produces a native image, the electromagnetic picture of the body**

Berger A,: Magnetic resonance imaging.
British Medical Journal MJ. 2002 January

Figure 71 Random directed Hydrogen protons are aligned in one direction during a Magnetic Resonance Imaging MRI
Own work

This alignment effect produces one order and one common sequence resulting in a clear picture of the body. In the course of MRI examination, the nano-magnets are activated by application of the radio waves. This causes a specific response. The strength of the cellular response depends on the water content in the different organs e.g. different images from heart being a strong muscle in comparison to the brain soft tissue.

MRI of the human brain coded in colours. Brain itself can decode the colours in a very special ways in the study mage by Bird C.M at al.

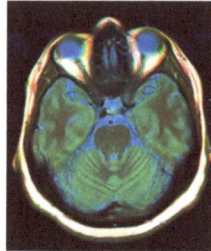

Figure 72 Colour coded visualization of MRI of the brain
Wikipedia Commons, by Nevit Dilmen

These modern studies on viral and bacterial communication confirm the pioneering research of Professor Luc Antoine Montagnier awarded with the Nobel Prize by in Medicine in 2008 for the discovery of the HIV virus by F. Barré-Sinoussi and Luc Montagnier and awarded in 2008 with the Nobel Prize for Physiology and Medicine. The documentary made with Professor Luc Montagnier by French TV in 2014 entitled *Water* memory https://www.youtube.com/watch?v=R8VyUsVOic0 went viral. My own clinical observation is that a diagnostic MRI scan can also be beneficial for specific conditions in its own right. If a diagnostic MRI scan is performed on patients who have been treated with medical acupuncture, especially patients with chronic inflammatory conditions such as Lyme disease or chronic fatigue syndrome, the improvement will often exceed the usual course of therapy and its outcome. This can be explained by recent scientific studies confirming that pathogenic bacteria communicate with each other via electromagnetic waves. A study published in 2016 by Dr Soghomonyan examines this remarkably interesting topic.

In 2016, at Princeton University's Department of Molecular Biology, Professor Bonnie Bassler confirmed the existence of bacterial communication via electromagnetic waves of water what was announced and described by Catherine Zandonella .

This new understanding of the electromagnetic nature of communication within our bodies gives us a better understanding of Greene's description of the vast electromagnetic universe we are living in.

New advances in quantum physics also reveal that superstrings can assemble and build huge membranes, which can be bent in space and constitute a living platform. Humans are attached to it via the force of gravity. These membranes are made from energized electrons or other subatomic particles. This is the basis of the multiverse theory, which says that more than one universe can exist in parallel. A huge membrane which is called "brane" can be an independent part of the universe. It could be connected to electromagnetic forces and ruled by its own gravity. The gravitational waves can hold more membranes, the brains in a specific position in the vast universe.

The gravitational waves necessary to hold the brain in space were sought by physicists. They searched for 80 years, since Einstein and Bohr predicted their existence. Finally, in February 2016, gravitational waves were detected https://www.theguardian.com/science/2016/feb/11/gravitational-waves-discovery-hailed-as-breakthrough-of-the-century.

6. The Human Heart's Morphogenetic Body Field

The electromagnetic body field is intangible, but it is powerful. It is mostly charged through heart and brain. It is a specific for every individual electromagnetic field of information, an invisible extension, an "extra" important shield for the human body. So, the human body like the entire Earth have an electromagnetic shield. Thu electromagnetic body shield and Erath's magnetic field interact with each other.

Pioneering research by the Institute of HeartMath Research Centre in California, USA brought some evidence to light of the morpho-genetic body field.

The body field receives and emits light and bio-photons, spiralling from and towards the human body. The bio-photons, the smallest quantum of light, are emitted from every living system. In medical research they can be detected as a specific biological electromagnetic radiation. The bio-photons that form the body field, along with elec-tromagnetic radiation are the signs of activity of the human heart, the DNA, the manifestation of the activation of our brain and other inter-nal organs.

Interconnected with Two Worlds

Human awareness allows every individual the realization of inter-connectedness with the Earth and direct environment as well as with the planetary system of the expanding galaxy. In fact outer space is closer than we think. It starts above the Kármán line at an altitude of 100 km above the earth. The Kármán line represents the boundary between the earth's atmosphere and outer space.

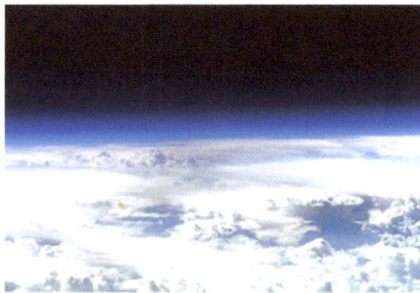

Figure 73 The Kármán line is beginning about 100 kilometres above the Earth. The Kármán line defines a boundary between Earth's atmosphere and outer space
Wikipedia Commons by NASA Earth Observatory

The universe is in effect two worlds in collision: One world of unimaginably tiny spaces and things – the quantum universe – and a world of vast space and events. Each of us needs to cross the intangible lines separating the invisible fabric of the Universe – the world of very small spaces – from the vast space above us. The space above us contains the sun, dark matter and exploding stars known as supernovas. If we want to mark our tracks in the future we have to access these opposite but complementary worlds of incredible, unlimited potentiality.

7. The Quantum Observer:
Living Probabilistically

The intelligence of the human heart can connect directly to the fabric of the Universe. Your cardiac intelligence will enable you to access the invisible world of quantum potentiality and you can live a new kind of life based on unlimited *probability of choices*.

The Quantum Observer

Medical physics has replaced Einstein's neutral and static observer. It was an unprecedented moment when science accepted the existence of a powerful quantum capability within each of us, the Quantum Observer (QO).

A Quantum Observer is a human being in a neutral position observing events or energy interactions.

We can all become influential Quantum Observers in regard to our own health. For the QO, the heart is an interface to the fabric of the Universe.

Healing requires the presence of a Quantum Observer and his/her undivided intention. Intentional observation collapses energized electrons, allowing them to release specific information which, when translated, re-enters 3D space-time causes intentional manifestations.

The Quantum Observer state is our gateway to the fabric of the Universe. This QO state is a heart-based oneness with the universe and is sometimes compared to the experience of swimming in the ocean of universal consciousness and intelligence.

Modern science and ancient wisdom agree that, if we are able to switch off our 3-D space-time preconditioned mind-set, the heart will connect to the fabric of the Universe, and we will enter a different, fully integrated dimension of perfect harmony. This entrance can happen during an experience of deep love and compassion, in state of meditation or prayer, during medical acupuncture treatment, Qi-gong, or in times of intense respiratory muscle training.

In this state of minimal mind interference, we can experience an exceptional reality: the invisible and intangible quantum reality, in which we are immersed. Being in this perfect state one can become a neutral, smart observer of actions happening inside of the body and at the same time outside, in the proxy and remote environment.

To be a knowledgeable QO, you need to understand heart/brain networking and their complex interdependence on each other. In fact the QO needs to develop a vision for the intelligent heart. The human heart is the "emperor" and the foundation of the living, holistic human body.

Medical physics defines the intentional actions directed to the electromagnetic field of our body as an intervention. It leads to a variety of manifestations and materializations in our 3D world, including perfect health, or illness. A crucial part of this intervention is the presence of a knowledgeable QO—and ideally that knowledgeable QO will be you. We all are designed to be the knowledgeable Quantum Observer and we can all the use intentional power contained in our metaphysical quantum heart.

The strength to access a pattern of health or to change the toxic pattern of disease can be amplified by teaming up with other Quantum Observers QOs. As an intentional QO you can push back from the manifested illness into the invisible 5th dimension of the fabric of the Universe.

The knowledgeable QO has conquered the inherited shortcomings passed to them via their DNA by consciously creating changes in their genetic code and its expression. He/she created a new epigenetics which is above the genetics. He/she can control the faulty potential of dormant genes and encrypted wrong information. This is important because, if somebody or something triggers a faulty gene, it can be dangerous enough to cause instant disease such a heart attack or even an immediate annihilation of the personality.

A knowledgeable QO is an expert in his/her individual health. Everybody has the potential to become an expert in own health. The QO can access the unlimited potential for healing contained in the fabric of the Universe. As the QO, you can put into practice a health-oriented quantum probability approach. Here are the things you need to engage with and understand to start to be a QO and to achieve a life of abundant health:

1. The fabric of the Universe as the source of unlimited potentiality for health
2. Medical physics as the science of light acting in the human body
3. Informational quantum entanglement of health and illness
4. The electromagnetic field surrounding the human body

Connected Hearts

When they fell in love a loving couple's hearts need to be connected. The heart of a child is deeply linked with its parents' hearts and the hearts of all individuals in a family. And it is interconnected with friends and with the global community. The heart of a leading scientist is connected with his/her collaborative research team and the heart of an employer with his/her employees. It looks like loyalty to a prosperous company, but the underlying framework is the connections between living and beating hearts.

The Heart-Brain Connection

The brain and mind oversee the functions of many internal organs and the anatomical functionality of the body including glands, bones, muscles, fascia, tendons and skin activity. They determine the correct coordination of kinetic, metabolic, hormonal and energy processes. The internal organs and the connective tissues are connected to brain and to each other via spine and spinal nerves innervating all parts of the body. The correct mapping of the body and the genes enables the operation of bodily awareness for an average life time of a human, now reaching to 80 or even 90 years.

The Electromagnetic 5th Dimension, the Fabric of the Universe

At the beginning of the 20th century Dr Theodor Kaluza, a Silesian genius mathematician, made a breakthrough in this matter. He was the first quantum scientist who solved Einstein's equations for general relativity for five dimensions, instead of four dimensions (3D plus time).

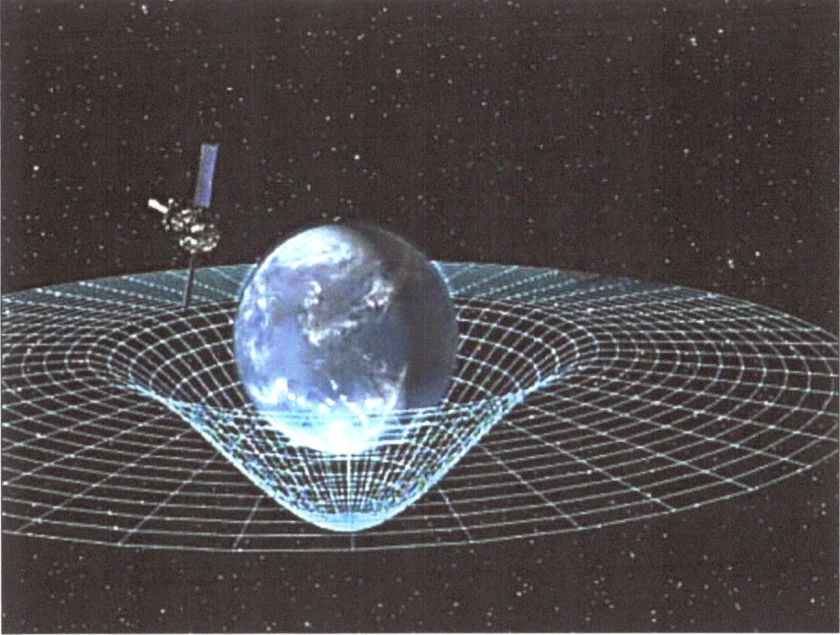

Figure 74 Artist concept of Gravity Probe B orbiting the Earth
to measure space-time, a four-dimensional description of the
universe including height, width, length, and time
Wikipedia Commons by NASA Public Domain

Einstein in his famous equation $E = MC^2$ concluded that mass (M) and kinetic energy (E) are equal, since the speed of light (C^2) is constant. The addition of the 5th dimension by Dr. Kaluza to Einstein's equation for general relativity produced the exact equation needed to describe electromagnetic fields. Kaluza was astonished to find that he could confirm scientifically the existence of a fifth electromagnetic dimension of the Universe using mathematical equations. https://en.wikipedia.org/wiki/Kaluza%E2%80%93Klein_theory

His work established the platform for the development of modern unified field research and made a solid foundation for the visible and invisible Universe, beyond Einstein's four dimensions 3D+time.

The 3D Universe described by Einstein includes the additional dimension of time flow, as the fourth dimension.

Kaluza sent a letter to Einstein describing his extraordinary discovery. Professor Einstein encouraged him to publish his work about five-dimensional space (5D reality including the electromagnetic field as the 5th dimension). Theodor Kaluza's discovery was published in 1921 in a paper, "Zum Unitätsproblem der Physik" (On the Unification Problem in Physics). https://www.worldscientific.com/doi/abs/10.1142/S0218271818700017

Kaluza's idea that four fundamental forces of nature (4FF) can be unified by introducing additional 5th electromagnetic dimension re-emerged much later as "string theory", developed from late 1960 to 1980. This theory attempts to explain the nature of the fabric of the Universe. String theory 1999 to 2008 was broadly discussed by Professor Brian Greene, American physicist, the founder of "The World Science Festival".

The theory suggests that the fabric of the Universe is built from very tiny vibrating strings in a single unified quantum field, in which 4FF (gravitation, electromagnetism, strong and weak nuclear forces) are active.

With the addition of the fifth electromagnetic dimension Dr Kaluza's theory was extended to Kaluza-Klein: the existence of black holes. According to this theory, the strings can build huge membrane structures in space (often abbreviated as "branes") a theory proposed by Toshiharu Nakagawa at al.

The Electromagnetic Field of the Human Body

The human body is a part of the three-dimensional Universe and has also its own, individual invisible electromagnetic field. This electromagnetic field is the result of the body's atomic structure and its water content. Water's hydrogen protons act as tiny nano-magnets, spinning always and producing an electromagnetic charge. The body field is mostly created by the heart, brain and the DNA of the human body. https://www.heartmath.org/research/

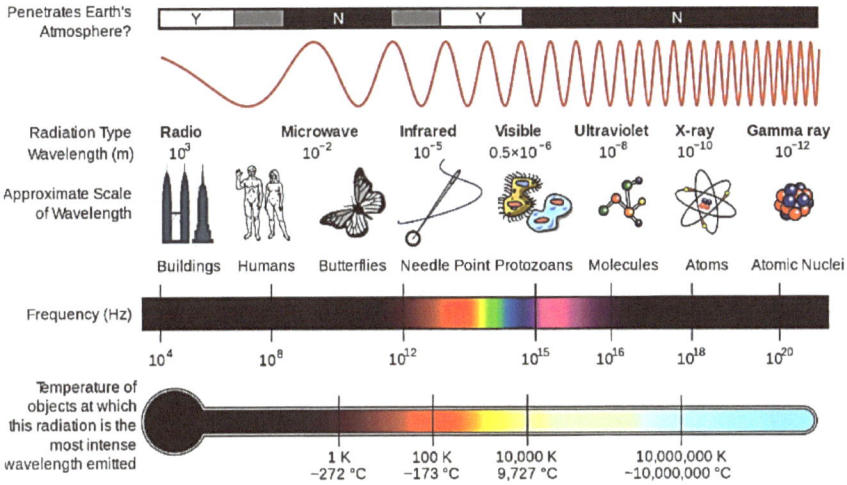

Figure 75 Interactions of organisms with electromagnetic fields from across the electromagnetic spectrum are part of bio-electromagnetic studies
Wiki Commons NASA - self-made information by NASA

Every molecule of water consists of two atoms of hydrogen and one atom of oxygen. Hydrogen's protons have a spin and they are constantly electromagnetically charged, acting as tiny magnets. The human body consists of about 70% of water, so it contains trillions of hydrogen protons acting as magnets. The constant charge produces energized electrons, which, in turn, create wave like movements in the human body. As a result, trillions of probability waves and immeasurable quanta of light form a stream of messages to our DNA.

The movement of trillions of energized electrons in the human body are the code of life, and unique to every human being. Probability waves usually manifest as DNA impulses, collapsed according to the pattern of metabolism or cardiovascular function.

And this results in heartbeats and the movement of respiratory muscles. The same energy moved by the intention of the Quantum Observer originating from a medical doctor, or a therapist can be used to repair the abnormal functional patterns of ill-health.

A good massage, a medical acupuncture session, correct physio-guidance or the advice of a medical doctor can improve damaged functionality. For example, a professional massage removes accumulated lactic acid from the muscles. Medical acupuncture accelerates a sluggish metabolism, supporting renewal and biological regeneration. The wise advice of a GP to use activated charcoal in case of diarrhoea can stop the growth of pathologic bacteria. The activated charcoal absorbs the toxins and restores good digestion and gastrointestinal functionality.

Two Views on the Quantum Observer Presented by Niels Bohr and Albert Einstein

The physicists Niels Bohr and Albert Einstein were both awarded the Nobel Prize in Physics, the highest scientific honour given to any researcher. They made great contributions to the development of quantum physics in the 20th century. However their views on the interactions of the Quantum Observer with the fabric of the Universe diverged significantly.

The major difference was their definitions of the Quantum Observer and its role in the quantum probability approach. A Quantum Observer is defined as a human being observing events or energy interactions from a neutral position. He/she is aware of the own intentions towards unfolding events. Bohr's holistic approach to QO considers a dynamic, influential human being who is sure of the unlimited potential of the fabric of the Universe – the power of one's own intensions. Bohr's QO is a knowledgeable person who can give rise to events from probability waves of the fabric of the Universe. Bohr's QO is aware of the forces connected to informational quantum entanglement acting at high speed even beyond the speed of light.

The QO in the meaning of Niels Bohr must overcome in his/her awareness the limitation of the speed of light set by Einstein at 299,792 km in a second. A smart Quantum Observer is also aware that information between people and systems is entangled and can be exchanged instantly. He/she knows about two main tools (heart/spirit) and (brain/

mind) which are able to explore and map 3D space-time, as well as the invisible fifth electromagnetic dimension. The brain/mind tool contributes to a comprehensive individual awareness.

Albert Einstein had a static view on the observer. He claimed that QO is not interacting with the Universe. The Universe in Einstein's view has no plasticity. Einstein's onlooker cannot make changes in the Universe; he/she simply passively looks at it from a non-executive position. Einstein's Quantum Observer can only measure certain features of the Universe. He also dismissed the internationally recognized concept of informational quantum entanglement, as it contradicted his own views. He expressed it in his famous sentence: *"Quantum entanglement is a spooky action at a distance."*

A smart QO knows about the heart/spirit tool and knows that humans are equipped with an instrument for exploring the invisible electromagnetic dimension. Perfect health results from a lifestyle of harmonious balance between both: the vital forces of the 3D space-time reality and the individual probability approach of the electromagnetic invisible field that we live in. This specific balance determines a successful, healthy life and longevity.

In fact, we can roam with our expandable mind in 3D space-time without physical limitations and through immeasurable long distances. We can exchange information instantly, quicker than at the speed of light, and receive quantum messages in a process known as intuition.

We know from experience, that a mother's quantum heart is connected with her daughter's heart. Even from 20,000 kilometres away a mother can instantly know her daughter's state of being. This connection is the essence of quantum entanglement and highlights the reality of borderless quantum communication which is not limited to 3D space-time reality.

One of the popular techniques useful for a skilled QO is meditation – an individual application requiring some knowledge and perseverance. Meditation can improve your breathing, and acts to reduce the mind's constant chatter, to accelerate healing.

The Second Quantum Observer

A skilled QO can observe him/herself or be observed by others. The person acting in the role of the second Quantum Observer (sQO) must be in a neutral position. The sQO might be a medical doctor, a friend, a family member. It can be an acupuncturist, a therapist, a physiotherapist, or a clinical psychologist.

Three Laws of Medical Physics

At the heart of 21st century medical physics are three laws. A closer exploration of these laws can help to determine the modern approach to healthcare and can explain the achieved results. Acting according to these laws will reward the QO with perfect health and will help the individual combat quantum illness.

The First Law: Unlimited Potentiality to Heal the Body

The knowledgeable QO can promote health, initiate the healing process and combat illness. The QO's solid intentions towards healing are the best weapon to fight illness, according to the quantum probability approach. The intentional QO can move energized electrons and direct them; he/she is able to understand big data, to transform it and apply the information to their own body.

The resulting intelligent message will change harmful energy patterns, and will improve and repair the functions and structures of the body. The chart above displays probability waves that are created by an unaccountable number of energized electrons. They have absorbed light (photons) and reached "superposition", the ability of a quantum system to be in multiple states at the same time until it is measured. This is the substance and the target for the healing intentions of the QO. The popular saying, "Where the attention goes the energy flows," is absolutely true.

Gaining Knowledge

A practical way to focus on your own healing is to gather information about how your body is doing, based on medical test results. This will strengthen your curative intention.

Pathology data needs to be assessed in detail. Initially this will be in a discussion with your health professional. Listen carefully to what they say. Take notes and ask questions. But there is usually a lot more information in these lab reports than the brief interpretation of your health professional, which was given to you. You need time and consideration to absorb their meaning – more time than the few minutes granted to you by your doctor.

Pluck up the courage to ask for copies of your lab test results, scans, ultrasound, etc. When you get home, read the report carefully and get onto the web and do your own research. When you feel you have a better grasp of things, meet with your health professional again and discuss treatment options or additional diagnostic procedures. If you're not comfortable, consider requesting a second opinion.

Sometimes it needs boldness to be assertive with health professionals, but it's your health that's at stake here and you should not be put off. If you feel daunted at the prospect of querying or challenging medical advice, it can help to bring a friend or relative along to the consultation. The simple fact of being outnumbered can make a difficult person more conciliatory. But also, you'll have an ally to speak with afterwards; they will have grasped some things you might have missed during the appointment, and that will add to your knowledge base.

Engaging in discussion will throw more light on the pathway to healing. In the process of knowledge accumulation, the QO gets valuable insights and will gain more understanding. This new knowledge and a more holistic understanding will convey beneficial messages and signals to your own DNA and begin the process of healing. Correctly identifying flawed processes in the body will produce positive impulses for improvement and cure.

Implementing the First Law

The activation of the first law of the unlimited potentiality for healing starts with an additional portion of energy absorbed by the complex bio-systems of the human body. The absorbed portion of energy will move the electrons into "superposition". An intensified 10 minutes abdominal breathing will increase the intake of oxygen. Gentle aerobic exercises, a hot drink, herbal tea infusions, warm clothing or hot sauna can be a good step in the right direction.

The situation of a single energized electron reflects that of groups of atoms, and a big aggregation of particles such as tissue, internal organs, and in fact to the entire human body in all its complexity.

After absorption of a quantum of light the energized electron moves to a higher energy level and inherits its special superposition. It makes a quantum leap and jumps into the invisible 5th electromagnetic dimension. Its movement is marked because, on its way back into visible reality, the electron emits a quantum of light, the smallest quantifiable amount of light, indicating its re-entry into 3D space-time reality.

The state of superposition gives an energized electron unlimited potential to move freely within the electromagnetic field of the hidden 5th dimension. The super-positioned electron is entangled with another electron, which is oriented oppositely. Both entangled electrons can freely exchange information at hyper speed. This includes information about their specific movements, their electromagnetic features such as spin and energy level. After delivering energy to the place where it was requested in the body, the electron becomes a carrier of new information from the hidden electromagnetic dimension which is necessary for healing according to the intention of the QO.

The Second Law: Quantum Entanglement

Quantum entanglement ("QE"), the second law of medical physics for healing, applies to any medical condition of the human body. According to medical physics QE is a "must". Any illness is intertwined with a healthy state and vice versa. Unhealthy entanglement involves a complicated situation from which it is difficult to disengage. The effect of quantum entanglement can be exponential in bringing health or illness to the body.

Quantum entanglement indicates that there is always the potential to restore health in case of illness. When applied to medical physics, the law of quantum entanglement determines both negative and positive health outcomes. If positive quantum events predominate, sound health will follow. Conversely, if the influence of the electromagnetic 5th dimension is generally negative – usually from negative interference from outside – eventually the signs of illness will manifest in the body.

In the context of medical physics, QE involves vast numbers of teaming electrons in the body, which interact in a much more powerful way than each particle could do alone. The intelligent pairing of electrons supports an instant exchange of energy and information, which is necessary to build a new pattern of functionality. After QE, the paired electrons in the human body cannot be described independently; they are totally interconnected. They are identical according to the information they contain, but oppositely oriented. We can compare them to the well-known, traditional Chinese medicine principle of yin/yang. They became totally dependent on each other and have formed an inseparable unit.

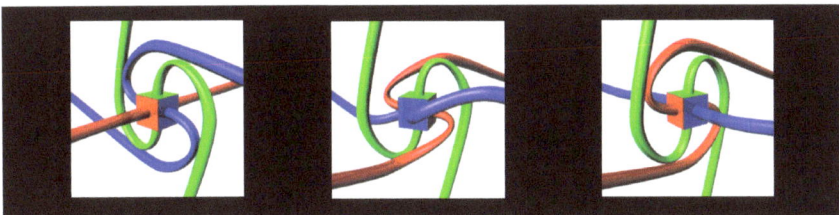

Figure 77 Entanglement
Wikipedia Commons by JasonHise

So, at the quantum level, health and illness are interchangeable. One sub-particle can be in 3D space-time reality and the other electron in the electromagnetic dimension of the fabric of the Universe. They can also be entangled one sub-particle inside and another outside of the human body.

The energized electrons form entangled gatherings, which are free and not limited by 3D space-time. One particle exists in the 3D reality and other paired particle exists in the 5th hidden dimension of the electromagnetic fabric of the Universe and they can rotate.

The entangled partners act as a unit and both parts of the pair are considered one in the same entity. The negative or positive orientation of the electron groups will then manifest in the form of health or illness.

Your Recovery

Your recovery depends on the level of your QO skills, and your intelligence and resilience against external hostile intentions. Additionally, the progress of healing is strongly influenced by the number of second Quantum Observers (sQO) you have around you. Their common accumulated knowledge will amplify the frequency of healing and it will eventually overcome the factors that led to the appearance of your illness in the first place.

The Third Law: Singularity

Enough engaged sQOs allied with your professional, medical Quantum Observers can amplify the frequencies of healing and result in *singularity*. The curative processes then become progressive, independent of the efforts of the QO. The collective efforts become totally fluid and frictionless. They will reach and pass the threshold, it will accelerate the momentum and it will result in an "explosion of healing".

One specific and persistent frequency of healing can activate the unlimited healing potential of the fabric of the Universe. An accumulation of healing energy, brought about through the acquisition of information, will strengthen your body's ability to overcome illness.

At the point when the electromagnetic field of healing is created, it is somewhat weaker than the old pattern which led to illness. A positive outcome depends on the complex actions you undertake and your determination to apply the attitude of QO.

The third law of medical physics, the singularity, is critical for healing. It is essential to support the cure until the singularity dominates your electromagnetic body field and reaches the invisible outer electromagnetic field of the fabric of the Universe.

A Single but Specific Frequency Can Dominate the Healing Process of the Body.

Healing is a search for the positive entangled twin of a negative disorder. This is the most essential part of the success. As a QO, you must be sure that any disorder can be cured. Regardless of the type or location of disease, the heart, liver, even the brain can be healed. The positive information supporting healing is in a superposition and waiting for the correct actions on order to be released. The patterns of health need a strong and repeated signal to amplify their frequency in 3D space-time reality. The necessary healing information is waiting to be energized, just like a single electron, and will re-enter diseased the body.

So, the affected body needs to be energized first. Your body must enter the higher frequency of healing. Then a healthy pattern will be awakened, ready to cross over from the electromagnetic quantum reality to the 3D reality of the body.

Quantum healing requires a totality of intention and constant focus on cure.

Your efforts and perseverance will make the curative field stronger. The total effective power of your healing frequency depends on your ability to find other smart, skilled Quantum Observers with the same unshakable intention for your cure. In deploying them, you will be able to reverse the reality of illness into a familiar pattern of health. Healing needs to engage specialists, therapists, family members and friends. They are connected to you via their intention.

For an example of a specific frequency dominating the entire unified field, think of a concert with great singer moving the crowds in excitement and unity. But the same energy can be achieved in a small workshop, for example, where many participants focus their attention on the speaker's narrative.

8. The Intentional Quantum Observer

Albert Einstein's idea of the static, unchangeable universe was shown to be flawed in 1982 with the results of the ASPECT experiment published in: http://www.drchinese.com/David/Aspect.pdf . The ASPECT trial confirmed that we all are all observers, communicating and interacting with a highly responsive and dynamic universe. Every knowledgeable and intentional QO influences the fabric of the Universe with unlimited potential. As a skilled QO, you're not limited to the biocentric model of the human body. You have access to the 5th electromagnetic dimension, and can bring together both the visible and unseen parts of the universe.

Acting as QOs, we can exchange information via quantum entanglement. Our growing awareness of our quantum entanglement with many humans, with our environment and the wider world, is part of achieving and maintaining sound health. We are also increasingly entangled with man-made artificial intelligence, which can sometimes constitute a negative factor for our health.

The quantum heart is a unique interface, connecting us with the invisible quantum reality of the fabric of the Universe. As humans we are in a privileged position to influence 3D space-time reality with our consciousness by directing our intentions towards it. The quantum heart can decode patterns of analogue information contained in the fabric of the Universe and translate it into new, health-giving energy patterns. As the intentional QO, you can master quantum reality and create according to the laws of medical physics. A true intention originating from the quantum heart opens the door to the quantum reality of the fabric of the Universe. Having focussed intention and an undivided mind enables us to reach the level of the superior mind, maintaining perfect health and acting for the benefit of mankind.

The Intentional QO Can Initiate the Cure from the Fabric of the Universe

Quantum physics discoveries revealed a very unusual landscape in our vast universe. Tiny sub-particles are changing their position into superposition all the time. They make quantum leaps and escape from our 3D space-time reality. Trillions of energized and super positioned electrons enter the electromagnetic 5th dimension every second and create a multitude of probability waves. The union of all these probability waves builds the fabric of the Universe and its unlimited potentiality.

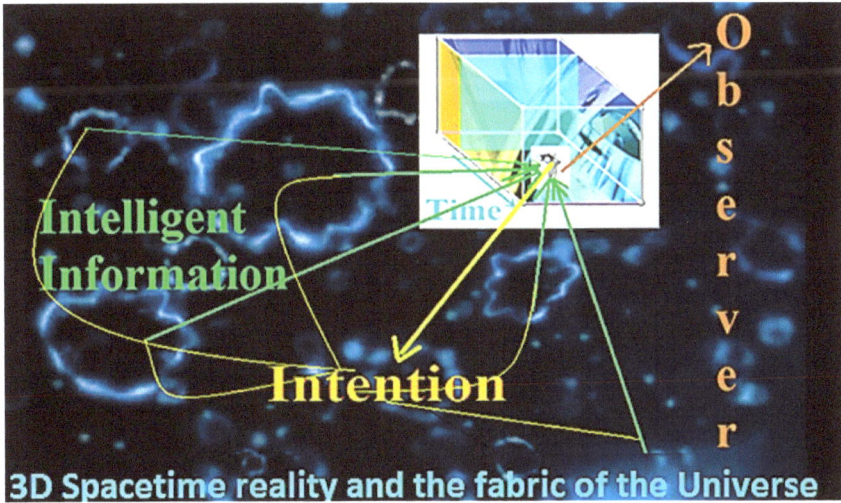

Figure 78 Relation between 3D reality and the fabric of Universe with the intention of a QO
Own work

Electrons dwell in their privileged superposition in the 5th electromagnetic dimension. They are not visible and cannot be detected with our eyes, nor even with the latest scientific tools. They are waiting for a

QO who, according to his/her intention, can collapse probability waves and manifest sound health. Swarms of sub-particles in superposition are ready to form the pattern of perfect health and to act to our benefit.

The moment they are observed, energized electrons lose their individual identity; they will assemble new configurations and build new information. The large amounts of data from the electromagnetic 5th dimension can interact with the electromagnetic field of the human body. The knowledgeable QO changes big raw data sets and transforms them into intelligent information. Once the intelligent information it translocated to 3D space-time reality it will be a driver for healthy energy patterns. As QOs, we can access the 5th electromagnetic dimension of the fabric of the Universe. In our quantum heart we are never limited. There is no limitation and there is no barrier to human consciousness.

The quantum heart and an individual human body interacting with the fabric of the Universe can process 70 to 80 million bits of information in a second. That is a lot of data. The human mind can perceive information at a limited speed of about 15 bits a second. The quantum heart and the quantum body can receive 5 million times more information in a second in comparison to our limited mind.

In the unlimited freedom of human consciousness everybody can move instantly, extremely far and to many locations. In fact, we can move to as many places as we wish. A skilled QO can even be in multiple places at the same time to perform health-oriented exploration.

During meditation, or in a moment of deep love, or a time of complete harmony, we can experience a state of congruence between the brain, the quantum heart and the quantum body. It is a state of minimal mind interference, and we can see the open door to the fabric of the Universe, the invisible quantum reality. In this unusual state we can access a different world, a world of perfection and of unlimited potentiality. In this bright world we can sometimes even glimpse upcoming future events and gather information and insights to help in making important decisions.

Sometimes this moment of profound insight appears to be a spectacular understanding of our interconnectedness and we can initiate the healing. Being immersed in this invisible reality we can hear and follow our divine calling; we can accelerate progress towards the fulfilment of our divine assignment. It all happens because we are practicing the highest level of focus on the quantum heart, connecting it to the fabric of the Universe, to its probability waves and to the eternal vibrating superstrings.

Your undivided and firm intention is a force that carries unimaginable amounts of energy. It can collapse trillions of energized electrons and can make a nuclear release of energy according to a specific, health-oriented configuration. Your utterly focused intention is an act of imprinting a specific pattern of intelligent information into the fabric of the Universe. It will produce sequences of informational movement for healing in your activated DNA.

The impacts of the intelligent information created by QO are like commands. They are able to transfer energy from the fabric of the Universe into 3D space-time reality, to bring about tissue repair and continuous regeneration.

A strong connection to the fabric of the Universe will produce an expansion of our consciousness and it will increase the intelligence of the quantum heart. And this in turn affects the active DNA. When the impulses have enough impact, they will uncover the true layers of our personality and help us to reach a higher level of holistic integrity, bypassing inherited "junk DNA".

The unlimited potential of probability waves makes it possible for an intentional action to assemble the energized electrons in two or more different places at once. Their re-entry into 3D space-time reality at two places at the same time is known as a bi-location. In your thoughts, as a QO, you can be in a different place than where you actually are. Most of us experience this many times in our lifespan.

Quantum Tunnelling

A phenomenon called quantum tunnelling reveals even more. Quantum tunnelling is the ability of electrons to pass through solid walls. With this miraculous power, electrons can escape from traps and pass through barriers that have been set up in space to hinder their movements. Less energized particles can borrow energy from the future to overcome a burden, such as a solid plate set in front of them. They behave highly intelligently, and this phenomenon can be reliably repeated. When they become sufficiently energized, they repay the energetic loan instantly.

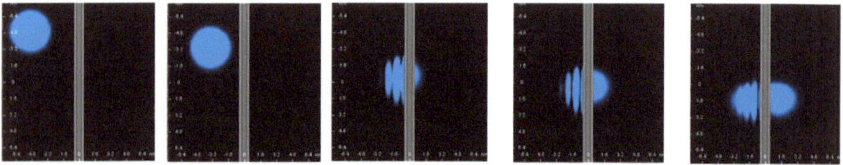

Figure 79 An energized electron passes through a barrier in an example of quantum tunnelling. An example of Tunnel Effect - The evolution of the wave function of an electron through a potential barrier
Wikipedia Commons by Jean-Christophe BENOIST at French Wikipedia

Our singular, undivided intention can direct probability waves. This process, when experienced and correctly understood, can restore health and change the quality of our consciousness. And this newly acquired consciousness will modify our future and throw light on past events, presenting them in the light of a new, holistic understanding.

Entanglement in Quantum Healing

The QO acts multi-dimensionally, and understands quantum entanglement. Two systems can have remarkably close informational/energetic relations. For example, two people who just fell in love can exchange information instantly and without any limitation in time and space. Our health and illness are entangled in the same way. The Quantum Observer's heart is able to tell which way she/he is entangled with illness and why it happened. The Quantum Observer needs to reflect and to realise why her/his connection to the unlimited potentiality for health in the 5th dimension of the fabric of the Universe has been temporarily restricted. Sometimes a QO can experience unusual responses from the fabric of the Universe to his/her mind directed actions. Things might turn out contrary to what is intended because the intention is not rooted in the heart. He/she needs to switch to pure intentions and to genuine quantum heart, which are completely different from cause and effect events that occur in 3D reality controlled by conditioned the mind.

The knowledgeable QO masters both 3D space-time reality of the mind and the invisible 5th electromagnetic dimension of the fabric of the Universe. The intelligent information and the underlying patterns of energy manifested in the 3D space-time reality can interact with the genes. Our DNA codes new sequences and the genetically sequenced information initiates any necessary repair, regeneration, and healing.

In 2004 Professor Michael E. Hyland published a breakthrough study focusing on the effects of a skilled medical QO on patient outcomes.

Hyland focussed on the therapeutic quantum entanglement that occurs between a patient and their therapist. This pioneering research explores an extended network generalized entanglement (ENGET) based on the complexity of systems and the laws of medical physics. The cornerstones of ENGET are:

- The role of the QO and quantum entanglement has evolved as a form of communication between people and can be used in healing.
- The human body is a complex and intelligent, self-organizing system.
- The body organizes itself to achieve genetically defined patterns, including bodily expression as well as specific lifestyle.
- The genes governing specific patterns and behaviour require positive feedback.
- Direct biofeedback is provided by quantum entanglement.

In his book, Dr Hyland argues that the optimal approach to healing includes three main components: lifestyle management, manual therapies, and psychological interventions. Furthermore, Hyland showed that these techniques are specific examples of quantum entanglement. Holistic therapy involves a subtle process of a patient being entangled with their therapist. The patient observes himself/herself and, through focused observation, he/she can learn and can become a more knowledgeable QO. The healing process, according to Hyland, is supported by physical remedies and a healing environment.

According to Hyland, quantum reality-based holistic therapy can create two kinds of informational field within the self-organizing network of humans, with two different outcomes:

- The network is not coherent enough for the patient to achieve healing, but a holistic therapeutic network can compensate for this and sometimes bring an improvement.
- A subtle holistic therapeutic field is strongly coherent, and it will guide the patient's self-organizing network to achieve healing.

Quantum Tunnelling and Its Role in Healing

Energized electrons, like all subatomic particles, have a quantum nature. They behave sometimes as waves and at other time as particles. As waves, they can "tunnel" through solid barriers. Quantum tunnelling is a key factor in many biological processes involving the breakdown of matter to energy, such as photosynthesis or cellular breathing. The reactions that allow energy to be extracted from molecules such as glucose, fats and amino acids follow the rules of quantum tunnelling.

Quantum tunnelling happens not only in our body but also in various types of modern technology. Quantum tunnelling is used in clothing industry to make smart, touchable membranes, like control panels within the ultramodern dresses. Quantum tunnelling technology can be found in mp3 players and in our mobile phones. It was used to provide fingertip sensitivity in NASA's Robonaut, human robotic development in 2012.

In 2000, Professor Nick Lane evaluated the role of quantum entanglement in mainstream medicine in the "The medical constraints on the Quantum Mind", published in the The Journal of the Royal Society of Medicine 2000; 93:571-575. He reviewed the laws of quantum physics and their relevance for medical sciences.

In his paper Lane discussed the guiding factors of quantum reality, quantum tunnelling and superconductivity. He assumes that tunnelling electrons cross the solid barriers of cell membranes to promote healing via intense and free information exchange. These free movements of electrons may also contribute to the fundamental mechanisms of our memory.

Medical Physics Is a Part of Holistic Medicine

Medical physics develops at high speed, complementing many other medical disciplines. It is part of holistic medicine.

In 1977 Doctors C. Norman Shealy, Gladys Taylor McGarey, Bill McGarey established the American Holistic Medical Association (AHMA), whose goal is to transform conventional healthcare into a more holistic model. They held that holistic medicine is an all-inclusive, integrated approach to medical practice, whereby all aspects of the patient's health should be taken into account; the individual should be treated and seen as a whole. And this includes addressing the patient's physical, spiritual, psychological, and social wellbeing.

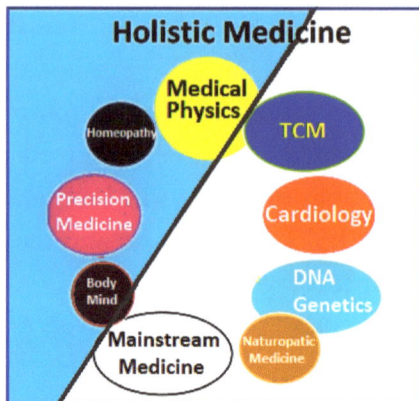

Figure 80 Major medical and natural
medicine disciplines building the
framework of the holistic medicine
Own work

Holistic medicine is an approach that fosters a cooperative relationship among all professionals engaged by a patient, leading towards the achievement of the patient's optimal physical, mental, emotional, social and spiritual health. It emphasizes the need to look at the whole person, including analysis of physical, nutritional, environmental, genetic, emotional, social, spiritual and lifestyle factors. It encompasses all stated modalities of diagnosis and treatment including drugs and surgery if no safer alternative exists. Holistic medicine focuses on education and personal responsibility, supported by the healthcare system, to achieve good balance and well-being. http://www.holisticmed.com/whatis.html

The scope of 21st century holistic medicine is spectacular. It starts with the probability approach to our body and the environment. It reaches into the vastness of space, to distant stars and galaxies, and all the way back into the interior of the quantum body. And the quantum body is another universe with unlimited potentiality, probability waves and the unified field of healing.

The spectacular dimensions of 21st century holistic medicine are put into focus in a stunning 3 minute YouTube clip by astrophysicist

Danail Obreschkow, *"The Science World Smiling Face Cosmic eye."* https://www.youtube.com/watch?v=haKMQBU5HVA

The term "quantum medicine" was used for first time in 1982 by William Nelson in the book "Subspace and Quantum Aspects of Biology", published by College of Practical Homeopathy, London. Professor Nelson's mathematical genius became famous through his calculations concerning the duration of oxygen supply for NASA astronauts and he saved the lives of the astronauts of the Apollo XIII Mission. The equations for the extraordinary situation in this spacecraft returning to Earth were so complex that nobody was able to solve them in the short time available. The astronauts landed safely on Earth within the calculated timeframe. By the time they landed, there was only 15 minutes' oxygen left. Nelson said,

"This quantum biology link will have several challenges for modern medicine, as it will not come to destroy the laws of medicine but will come to fulfil them. We will start to understand that there are different systems of medicine that evolve from our more exact system of biology.

He continued, "The implications of this will tend toward naturopathy, homeopathy and energetic medicine techniques ... We welcome the reader to an exciting psychological challenge to develop the mind and to reach beyond the paradigms of a synthetic, pharmacological, chemical society into a more deeply-based, reverent, and exact system of quantum biology and quantum medicine".

In the diagram are displayed the major applications building the framework of holistic medicine. The diagonal line separates two different approaches to holistic medicine.

The first approach is displayed in the white field. It contains the components of holistic medicine operating in 3D space-time reality. The components in the blue field involve the probability approach, existing within the electromagnetic body field and the fabric of Universe within the human body.

The application of medical physics creates a new understanding of the healing process that focuses on a vigilant and knowledgeable Quantum Observer. The QO's curative intention is in the context of modern and holistic medicine. This focused intention has unlimited potential for healing within the spectrum of natural and mainstream medicine.

9. Quantum Health

The heart is a source of healing and regeneration. It is the foundation of intellectual wellbeing.

The main pre-condition to achieving perfect health is the fusion of the awareness operating in 3D space-time reality with the 5th invisible dimension, the exploratory field of consciousness. This is the key to understanding our life and our divine assignment on planet Earth. The divine assignment is specific to everyone. The practice of evidence-based, 21st century medical physics considers the interactions between solid 3D reality with the original intention placed of the fabric of the Universe. It needs skill because it goes beyond our usual perception. At the end, this specific ability will determine our lifespan and our state of health.

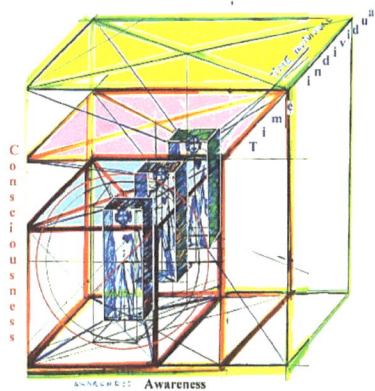

Figure 81 Relationship between 3D
reality + time and the awareness and
consciousness of an individual
searching for healing and health
integrity
Drawing by Angela Rudhart-Dyczynski

The quantum heart and the human body are made from vibrating atoms and their sub-particles, electrons and photons. The human body has electromagnetic features because of the vast number of the Hydrogen protons constituting the major component of the body's H_2O. It contains probability waves, with their unlimited potential for health. The human body, governed by the quantum heart, is a source of intelligence which is the driving force for a constant process of renewal and transformation.

It is not easy in the modern world to be single minded, and entirely focused on healing. However we were born with an integrity that includes perfect health. Quantum health and holistic healing are a one-directional and intentional process with a one-way ticket. Our "Yes" to health and to a healthy way of life can never be questioned.

To achieve the curative singularity, and to stay focussed on a healthy lifestyle can be lifesaving. Here are your priorities for health:

1. Be a receptive and knowledgeable QO.
2. Be trained in diaphragmatic breathing and practice respiratory muscle training every day.

3. Find a trustworthy partner, your second Quantum Observer.

4. Have an outdoor lifestyle and be exposed to sufficient natural light and sunshine.

5. Perform regular self-health checks and apply biofeedback daily.

6. Drink good quality water. Water carries vital information for health and is an abundant source of bio-available minerals, which cannot be substituted by any other drink.

7. Understand the healing power of analogue frequencies and practice healing sounds. Listen to birds, sing a song and play music; listen to the ocean or contemplate nature in the wild.

8. Apply the rules of epigenetics and transform your body shape, using oxygen-based exercises, walking with abdominal breathing, doing intermittent fasting, practice qi- gong, yoga or meditation

9. Fast intermittently. Use precious vegetables such as fennel, beetroot, sweet potatoes, cauliflower, yam and broccoli; use healthy spelt grain; consume sufficient fruits; and drink fresh pressed fruit daily. A cold pressed juice would ideally be pineapple with lemons or carrots with ginger. During fasting intervals, follow the Hollywood diet consisting of cold pressed fresh pineapple juice and liquids such a coffee, water or tea.

10. Minimise stress and your exposure to coronavirus and other respiratory viruses with herbal teas, plants such as artemisia vulgaris (Mugwort) artemisia absinthe (sweet Wormwood) or artemisia annua, aloe vera, and herbal tinctures such as Swedish bitters.

11. Regularly boost your immunity with acupuncture treatment, remedial massage therapy or foot reflexology.

12. Love and enjoy the precious gift of life with its kindness and all-inclusiveness. We are part of the planet Earth and we have borrowed our quantum body from it.

Quantum Illness

In every disease, we face a disordered quantum heart; a strange reality of illness engulfs us. It appears slowly or instantly in our 3D space-time, the mind mapped reality. It appears in our lifetime although we do not want it. We are increasingly aware of the symptoms and slowly decode their deeper meaning. The normally friendly fabric of the Universe turns upside down and seems now to be our challenger. The new circumstances are characterised by suffering and an unexpected low quality of life.

The usual healthy holistic state of the self-organizing body does not match the perfect health potential contained in our DNA. The reality sinks far below our expectations. We face completely opposite conditions to those of the perfectly working health fundamentals well known to most of us. We are catapulted into an unhealthy and strangely distorted dimension.

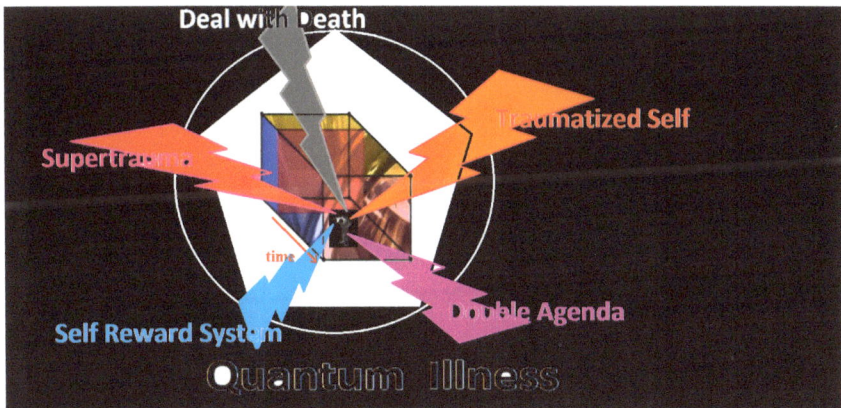

Figure 82 Five components of Quantum Illness: 1.Traumatized Self 2. Self Satisfaction 3. Double Agenda 4. Deal with Death 5. Supertrauma
Own work

Prior to the manifestation of quantum illness in 3D space-time something relevant has happened in the invisible fabric of the Universe and it has impacted the electromagnetic field of the heart and the entire body. Toxic information has scrambled the invisible electromagnetic body field. This is the major negative action coming from outside. Why it does happen? Everybody is born into a specific family bondage. The integrity of a child can be easily invaded. More often someone takes away the child's developing independence and binds it to a manipulative field. This happens for a reason; usually the underlying intention is to exploit the child's life force.

A child who is conditioned in early childhood has to deal with the malicious impact of the invader. This malign force can make an imprint or even a hole in the invisible shield of the child's electromagnetic body. As a result it can react with the development of three major elements of quantum illness: traumatized self, self-rewarding system and the operational double mind. The person of two minds has a hidden agenda, the behaviour that is not openly admitted or known or visible at the surface, insincere to the own personality. Later in life, as a teenager or a young adult, a deal is done with death. The immature traumatised person signs a contract which includes an option of killing – the further action of a traumatized self. This is the fourth component of quantum illness and can make the growing individual vulnerable to attacks towards her/his integrity. At this stage the affected teenager or young adult desperately needs healing; otherwise he/she will face a supertrauma, the fifth component of quantum illness.

If an ill individual does not receive support in the course of a quantum illness, he/she will never stand up and change the toxic circumstances. Then the oppressing illness and corrupted information patterns will disrupt, fragment and destroy her/his health. The cure lies in the development of the attitude of a Quantum Observer. A child or a teenager needs supervision; they need genuine insights and a solid level of knowledge through long lasting support.

When sickness arises, four components of quantum illness can be identified. They are the reason for the appearance of quantum illness in 3D reality. The fifth component, supertrauma, is a final effort on the part of the Universe to heal the person from quantum illness.

1.   The Traumatized Self

The first component of the quantum illness, the traumatized-self can be easily identified by taking a moment to look back and reflect on your early childhood.

There is a chain of events leading back to the appearance of the quantum illness. Take a moment to build a timeline and find the first component of the quantum illness. Looking back to early childhood, almost everybody will discover not only one but many traumas.

Anyone who has reached adulthood has experienced suffering in early life. These traumas affected the heart, the body, the soul, the mind and the spirit/conscience. They scrambled the electromagnetic body field, made a malicious imprint or even a hole in it. A damaged invisible body shield then exposes the body to the influence of the destructive intelligence of disease.

The relevant traumas can include: a cold parent, missing unconditional love, violence at home, medical procedures, violating child's independence, punishments or abuse. The child's suffering has not been understood and not recognized by its family. Traumatic impacts have made an imprint in the heart and in the electromagnetic body field and have impacted the child's developing consciousness.

This is a big mystery. How it is possible that a human being's unlimited potential for health can be altered and reduced through the traumatized-self. What moves a pure child to develop toxic self-satisfaction? And what factors allow a child's innocent mind to be contaminated by the hidden double agenda?

Many of the triggering factors for a traumatized self can be found in the Yoga Vasistha – a famous, influential Hindu text. The book The Supreme Yoga is a new translation of the Yoga Vasistha. https://www.booklibrarian.com/pdfepub/yoga-vasistha-free-pdf/

Under the date of 12 January at the page 19 we can find the words of the wise sage Rama. This is a quote related to traumas in childhood:

"Even childhood, the part of life which people ignorantly regard as enjoyable and happy, is full of sorrow. Helplessness, mishaps, cravings, inability to express oneself, utter foolishness, playfulness, instability and weakness, all these characterise childhood. The child is exposed to countless happenings around it; they confuse the child and arouse various fantasies and fears. The child is impressionable and is easily influenced by wicked-ness. In consequence the child is subjected to control and punishment by its parents.

Though the child may appear to be innocent, the truth is that all sorts of defects, antisocial tendencies and neurotic behaviour lie hidden and dor-mant in it. When the child goes to school, it receives punishment at the hands of teachers, and all this adds to its unhappiness.

When the child cries, in order to pacify it, its parents promise to give it the world and, from then, the child begins to value the world, to desire worldly objects."

The Concise Yoga Vasistha was translated by Swami Venkate-sananda, and published in 2010, SUNY Press, please compare the page 14.

The above cited quote illustrates the impacts shaping the trauma-tized self. A child's unlimited creative potential finds an unhealthy way to deal with traumas. One way is the establishment of a personal self-sat-isfaction system. This is the second component of the quantum illness.

2.   Self Satisfaction

The self-satisfaction of a child with a traumatized-self does not know borders and it has no limitations. It has a motto: "Get it, whatever it takes."

It becomes a habitual attitude. Repeated self-satisfying acts over-write the healthy information contained in the coding DNA.

In years, the first three components of the quantum illness produce fragmentations and divisions in an affected person. It can already cause the development of a fragmented identity. When the personal self-satisfaction system touches on social or sexual taboos it needs to be untraceable. The child adopts a different face to the family and social environment, and a different attitude towards personal and self-invented rewards. The success of a personal self-satisfaction system can only endure when it is kept secret; and this is no problem for the unlimited creative potential of a child. The child develops a double agenda, which is the third component of the quantum illness.

3.   Double Agenda

The traumatized self wants to escape to a better place, to a realm that is invisible to others. It develops a double mindedness also known as a double agenda. The person of two minds learns that telling lies is a way to achieve its desired reward. It lies also because of fear.

The child fears parents, siblings and other family members invading its private space. The double agenda has to satisfy their controlling attitude, the challenging demands of the social environment and the child's self-satisfaction system. The child may find a way to access its immature sexuality.

Sexual self-satisfaction as the intended self-reward can be a significant driver of the double agenda. It can create shame, guilt and can weaken general health. It can reinforce the secret world of taboos and produce a need to conceal. It can add to a child's emerging sexuality an abnormal background.

Double agenda is a not a positive strategy. It oscillates between matter and anti-matter, between life and death. In brings contradictory messages to the fabric of the Universe. Over time the child becomes used to contradictory messages and it has fully coded the double agenda in its DNA. The false information goes into every cell, and contaminates the heart, brain and other internal organs.

The double agenda has no limits and leads to manifestations of quantum illness in 3 D space-time reality. In a progressive, aggressive form, double agenda ends with death or self-termination. Double agenda always make a way in our defence system for the dark forces and destructive intelligence of illness.

Repeatedly applied double agenda as an internal strategy overwrites the DNA in meaning of epigenetics and it becomes a part of the individual's DNA. It is tolerated and hidden for a long time, resulting in fragmentations of the personality. The fragmented identity of the traumatized-self is always ready to take risks to achieve its desired self-satisfaction.

One of the strategies to reach a feeling to be awarded can be excessive buying. Self-awarding in our modern times known as the retail therapy, where the primary purpose is to improve buyers mood and to satisfy the pathologic drive originating from the traumatized self. The name retail therapy is ironic acknowledging that shopping hardly qualifies as true therapy in the medical or psychotherapeutic sense.

It was first used in the 1980s, with the first reference being this sentence in the Chicago Tribune of Christmas Eve 1986: "We've become a nation measuring out our lives in shopping bags and nursing our psychic ills through retail therapy." Schmich, Mary (24 December 1986). "A Stopwatch On Shopping". Chicago Tribune according to Wikipedia: https://en.wikipedia.org/wiki/Retail_therapy

The traumatized-self operates at a higher level of pathology. It can rage, offend and produce insane violence to get a desired reward at all costs. It takes risks for the desired rewards, even if the process can end with death. If any opportunity approaches, it has no objection to taking even a deadly risk.

Everybody's life is progressing in 3D reality according to their personal timeline. Almost without exception we have incorporated in our childhoods the three components of quantum illness: the traumatized-self, the double agenda and the self-reward system. Every individual carries the components of quantum illness into adulthood and at some stage the traumatized-self makes a deal with death. And this is the fourth component of the quantum illness.

4.   The Deal with Death

The deal with death could be an acceptance to kill other humans; maybe an agreement to eliminate an older family member or an unborn child. It may be forced by circumstances; for example a decision to agree with abortion. The deal with death is a situation in which, under pressure of medical authorities, we make a decision to switch off the life support for a child or a loved one.

In a very simplified form a deal with death could be a reverse mortgage, in which somebody accepts his/her own death as a part of financial loan and agrees to certain conditions. A deal with death in everyday life could be manipulating your last will as an instrument of pressure on your family and loved ones.

Another example of a deal with death may be supporting somebody to "Die with Dignity". Or it might be signing on to a militant organization or intelligent service, or to become an unmanned military drone pilot, equipped with missiles and kill lists. Or you might become a double agent in an intelligence service with a licence to kill. A deal with death sometimes takes a hybrid form. It looks good and attractive from one side but on the other side it will bind an individual to a lethal commitment. Deals with death proliferate in modern life and take the form of contracts, commitments and obligations. It has almost an unlimited potential to appear in one form or another, to mislead an individual to sign a deadly agreement. It leads into an abyss where the individual is exposed to a negative chain of reactions and a hostile attack. In this abyss nobody can cushion the impact of the approaching supertrauma. In choosing to operate predominantly in the 3D space-time reality the individual diminishes the development of consciousness and can aggravate the symptoms of quantum illness.

The killing technologies of the 21st century are developing relentlessly, harnessing the unprecedented precision of artificial intelligence. There is more to come; killer robots are on the way to dehumanize the process of killing altogether. We are approaching a world where an individual name merely needs to be added to a kill list, and the AI apparatus of the state will look after the rest. The condemned victim will be tracked down and terminated without further human intervention.

The deal with death can lead to the development of a "killer personality" or it might end in suicide.

The life of a person with the four components of quantum illness can progress seemingly well, despite the many levels of manipulation and lies necessary cover up the double mind and the self-satisfaction – unless it is impacted and complicated through the occurrence of the fifth component, the supertrauma.

5. Supertrauma

The heart became a battlefield. The quantum body and the "elephant mind" can manage the four components of quantum illness for a long time, especially when the individual is skilled in acting according the double agenda. Why not accept it, when today governments work perfectly to this principle? However there comes a time when the traumatized-self overflows with the amount of false, toxic data that it has to manage. The person with quantum illness loses control and starts making bad decisions. This precondition opens the way for a supertrauma.

The time prior to a supertrauma can be very stressful, confusing, and even weird. Just before a supertrauma event, the fabric of the Universe urges the affected person to stop the double agenda and the self-satisfaction system, to protect their health and to restore the balance, to rebuild the strength of the electromagnetic shield. Otherwise the illness progresses and it can catapult the individual to the next step, an irrevocable state of quantum illness.

A supertrauma can accelerate a seemingly simple common cold to a severe illness due to unexpected complications. It can manifest as a Coronavirus infection and even crash the person, who is too busy to manage the spiral of double agendas, self-satisfaction systems and the deals with death. A person can become so busy with compensation of the four other components of a quantum illness that she/he can lose access to the full intelligence and awareness of 3D space-time reality. Their decisions and judgments become more and more biased. And this sets the stage for the approaching supertrauma.

The supertrauma is very individual and has a wide variety of manifestations. It can be a big material loss. It can manifest as a loss of social values such as dignity, freedom or human rights. It can appear as an accident or stroke with loss of bodily independence, or as a heart attack.

It can be a car accident with a spinal cord injury, or a tragic loss of loved ones. More simply, it might be a crisis in an unhappy marriage. It can be a situation of a grown man who should be a father behaving like a child, because the traumatized-self of his childhood has not healed. It can be a killing or abuse in the family inner circle or a death in a terrorist attack against civilians.

Sometimes the supertrauma can have an aura prior to the main event. The supertrauma comes unexpectedly, like a thunder-storm, and cannot be prevented. It cuts a hole in the electromagnetic shield of the impacted person. Sometimes it can be felt like a laser light impact or an electromagnetic hot shower in the vulnerable human body. It ruptures the electromagnetic shield, the guardian of quantum health, leaving it exposed to the dark forces of destructive intelligence. Now, the destructive intelligence of illness has free access to your life force. It can damage the heart and the quantum body. It compromise awareness, the ability to navigate in 3D reality and significantly limits the spiritual level of consciousness. It can invade your quantum entangled family members or friends.

A supertrauma will bring an individual to the frontier between life and death. There is no escape from it. A supertrauma is never sequenced as a cause and effect event because it comes from the invisible, from the fabric of the Universe and it appears as a strange event in 3D space-time reality. From the 3D space-time perspective, a supertrauma appears as a random and usually unpredictable tragedy. It is non-linear and can be exponential in its violence. It has a devastating impact on your life and quantum body.

The supertrauma usually follows a deal done with death. More about justice in 21st century can be found on author's blog: https://justice696334899.wordpress.com/

Quantum Illness Relates to Quantum Justice

In this age of proliferating challenges, disruptive technologies, grim reaping, digital wildfires, societal "runaway collapses", destabilising feedback loops and systemic breakdowns, many of our established values have been radically changed. Our social commons and human values are degraded by the proliferating weeds of artificial intelligence (AI). Low level algorithms are slowly choking not only the performance of the internet but also our modern life.

Polarised positions harden the modern world into a winner-takes-all contest. The interactions of disruptors slow down the execution of justice. The pursuit of justice requires enormous effort and seems to lead more often to a physical confrontation.

Justice is no longer a linear process by which fairness and law are administered. It does not progress in 3D reality according to expected timelines. The justice system delivers wild and unexpected outcomes. Justice causes individual clashes and it doesn't act according to the rules of cause and effect. It demands from an individual a firm stand in the arena of law with numerous flash-points of intervening and destabilising forces. Justice has become a costly process of personal and spiritual development; however it leads always to the expansion of our consciousness.

As the pace of change accelerates, a fair justice is not simply provided by a court or government agency. Justice in the 21st century is primarily a personal interaction with the invisible quantum reality of the fabric of the Universe; it is truly a personal challenge. Sometimes a seemingly unjust response bounces from the fabric of the Universe, from the depths of interconnectedness, unexpectedly revealing your own double minded intentions. Quantum justice appears in 3D space-time reality with unpredictable force to hit those individuals violating the laws of the Universe. The justice-related quantum response is generally rapid and nonlinear.

Nobody can escape justice-related challenges. Independent of the age, gender or the ethnic heritage the Universe forces everybody to act as knowledgeable individuals. You might be 85 years old or 16, and wondering why life has fallen so far short of expectations.

There are two critical factors of negative interference causing this unexpected response from the fabric of the Universe:

1. Operating in 3D space-time reality most of your life
2. The appearance of a Quantum Illness as a response to the violation of the laws of the fabric of the Universe

Operating in 3D space-time reality most of your life

Considering the diagram below can be helpful in classification of the own positioning in the present moment of reading those pages.

The 3D reality occupies a unique position in everybody's life. It is displayed in the lower/right part of the diagram below. The model of the 3D reality only is too simple to explain the complexity of lives and the challenges we as humans face so the diagram displays also the electromagnetic, invisible fabric of the Universe accessible by heart and spirit.

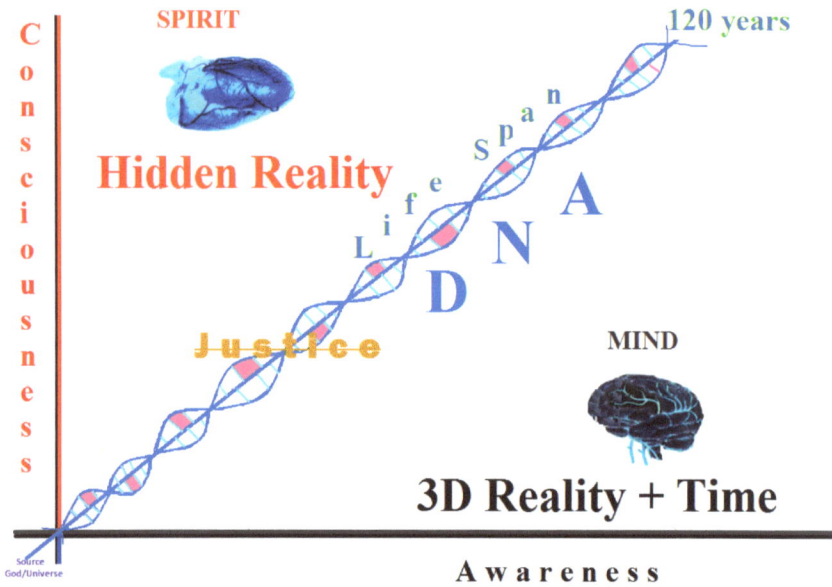

Figure 83 Relation between awareness, consciousness and justice in a life span of an individual
Own work

Consciousness is displayed in the upper left. It is poorly explored and almost unknown to many of us because it is invisible to our general senses and 3D oriented perception. The importance of consciousness is not easy to comprehend as most of us go through life without the benefit of good teachers and experienced spiritual advisers.

The dividing line in the middle of the diagram is your living DNA, which can be programmed for a short or long life span (up to 120 years).

The lower part is the domain of awareness. This is the realm of daily reality, of which we are most aware; we understand how it works.

The mind calibrates the 3D world and usually maps the 3D space-time reality correctly. It calculates all events, facts and occurrences in the physical world and produces the grid of awareness. This 21st century generation knows how to produce the grid of awareness: to use a car, computer or smart phone. Some people are masters of 3D space-time reality and they model it perfectly, achieving amazing financial and social outcomes.

The upper/left part of the diagram shows the hidden reality, the fabric of the Universe, the domain of consciousness. It is invisible but, at same time, when it comes to justice it is very powerful. In the domain of consciousness we have the beating, intelligent heart and the invisible spirit as the tools for engaging with reality beyond 3D. The virtually mapped grid constitutes our conscience.

From this perspective your life span is intimately connected with awareness and consciousness. Maintaining equilibrium between those two components is essential to a long and just life. A balanced long life will develop knowledge and wisdom and expand the frontiers of consciousness. The aim is to progress in a balanced life according to the DNA mid-line. But as individuals we face the opposite forces trying to bring us away from the balanced middle line. To maintain the balanced life you must to defend yourself and experience the issues of justice.

Consciousness of justice was and still is a must for each of us. It is only a question of time; a critical situation will appear in 3D space-time reality and demand that we act according to quantum justice.

The Existence of a Quantum Illness

Almost everybody has a quantum illness, just as almost everybody has a heart or spine disorder. Only the extent of impairment varies. Sometimes the tipping point will be reached and your survival will depend on making the right decision.

We can model this in three different ways. A person with a quantum illness might still have not experienced a supertrauma. Another individual can dwell just at the frontier between a normal life and a strange reality caused by a supertrauma. Another might be just at the cusp of catastrophe and have a premonition of a supertrauma.

Healing Quantum Illness

Quantum healing is a hybrid war within the heart affecting the mind and the whole body. It is a clash between the mind, which is overloaded with 3D space-time information, and the heart which is rooted in the quantum reality of the fabric of the Universe. It is a fight between concepts placed in the conditioned mind and the exponential, sometimes miraculous powers of the quantum reality. It is also a battle between reactive emotions arising from generational junk DNA, and the cool Quantum Observer's determination for healing.

Quantum illness can produce a variety of disorders including:

- depression
- suppression of the immune system
- autoimmune disease
- chronic fatigue syndrome
- atrial fibrillation
- stroke
- heart attack
- sudden cardiac death
- cancer
- overweight
- ulcerative colitis
- eczema of the skin
- obesity
- diverse addiction
- drug abuse
- a variety of sexual abnormalities.

These are just some examples. The full list is much, much longer.

When the protective electromagnetic shield is breached by harmful information, the body will manifest an illness in 3D space-time reality. And this results in the many painful, frustrating and bothering symptoms.

The most severe form of quantum illness is a supertrauma, where the impacted person is catapulted to the frontier between life and death. The effects of a supertrauma can be reversed, but only through the strong determination of the affected person to persevere in restorative health protocols. They also need the advice of many medical professionals, and the support of family and helpful, assertive friends.

In the case of a supertrauma something unusual has happened to the balanced state of health. Something caused the destructive forces of illness to crack down on the individual's immunity and the self-organizing system of a healthy body. There are many possible causes, such as poor health advice encouraging risky actions, or a mighty suppression of the body's electromagnetic field through some modern electronic technology.

Sometimes a 21st century business model supported by artificial intelligence can be a cause or a contributing factor. These exploitative business models are admired as being alive and health-promoting, but they are not.

Digital technologies and virtual business models are new forces that limit the freedom of an individual. This is the toxic secret of digital technology; it is a new way to undermine health awareness in the modern world. These man-made tools can cause imbalances and push a healthy person to take unhealthy, even lethal, risks, entering a field of chaotic, contradictory information. If you become too taken up with digital technologies it can trigger quantum illness.

Personal stress and informational overload can add to quantum illness, causing disease, infection or injury. Sometimes, through their strong interference, external forces will change the initial intentions of an individual and produce destructive chaos leading to disaster.

Only comprehensive knowledge and proven wisdom from the perspective of the Quantum Observer can bring an effective shift and can push back against these malign forces.

The timeline of a quantum illness is usually a long, developing worst case scenario. But the final supertrauma can appear suddenly. A quantum illness has strong components that impact your health and life force. Only a vigorous response can stop and to reverse the direction.

Double Agenda

The cause of our quantum illness is the double agenda we adopted at a very early age. As a knowledgeable QO you will undertake targeted actions to stop the double agenda.

The double agenda contaminates DNA and becomes part of the personality of the affected person. It needs courage to stand up and to change the double agenda. It requires smart, heart based decisions and iron perseverance. A knowledgeable QO will not be struck down, stunned and paralysed through the 3D space-time perception of quantum illness but will take the necessary appropriate steps to re-establish balanced health.

Healing will never happen as long as the brain is caught in a double agenda scheme. A double agenda will always produce a zero effect in the quantum field because it sends contradictory messages to fabric of the Universe. The result is no response from the Universe. The double agenda greatly limits the unlimited potentiality for the health creation.

You are the only carrier of your own holistic sensitivity and health-oriented sensibility. To become a QO, you must regain your trust in the unlimited potential of the quantum heart to restore full functionality. The quantum heart can help to extract life-giving information from mind-rooted, pre-programmed and digitally oriented information and biased perceptions.

Quantum illness is a not an incurable disease. It is a reversible functional state. It needs holistic and intentional actions to push damaging information back to the electromagnetic dimension of the fabric of the Universe, where it came from.

The Curative Actions of the QO and the Dominant Role of the Quantum Heart in Healing

When faced with illness, the smart QO immediately comes back to the incredible potential of the quantum heart, confident of its unlimited potential for healing. The knowledgeable QO knows that holistic health is governed by the quantum heart and its intelligence. The quantum heart inherits enormous potential for holistic healing and self-renewal.

The heart is linked to the limitless potentiality of the invisible, electromagnetic 5th dimension and the potentiality of probability waves. In initiating healing, the QO connects to the guiding force from within. Every heartbeat electrifies the DNA in every cell. It activates renewable healing information contained in the DNA for perfect health. The heart is a source of healing, regeneration and the foundation of intellectual wellbeing.

The Quantum Observer's solid and undivided intention is fundamental for the restoration of good health. An absolute single-minded focus on the topic of healing is like a laser light illuminating the darkness of the quantum illness. This light will burn away unhealthy information contained in the generational junk DNA and can uncover temporarily darkened, methylated genes.

A skilled QO will develop a solid, unshakable intention for healing and influencing both 3D space-time reality and the electromagnetic dimension of the fabric of the Universe. The intentional QO can listen to the intelligent heart. When the process of gathering knowledge and wisdom reaches a critical level, it will produce a quantum leap to singularity, and initiate unstoppable healing.

The QO must know that quantum illness can produce any kind of heart disorder, heartaches, palpitations, abnormal heart rhythm or even broken heart syndrome. The quantum illness came into existence in 3D space-time reality because of violations of the laws of the fabric of the Universe.

The QO should be stable as a rock and firmly rooted in the knowledge that a positively charged and healthy pattern of health is waiting, ready for re-awakening in the electromagnetic 5th dimension of the fabric of the Universe.

Threatened by unpleasant symptoms and bad signs, depressed by the darkness of suffering, one can become locked up in the box of pathology. It looks like you have no key to unlock the oppressive box. You become totally focused on diseased 3D space-time negativity. Some people will even accept the descent into quantum illness. They come to think of it as part of the aging process and even become attached to their illness because it brings a rewarding increase in social or familial attention. But the skilled QO will disconnect from all limitation of 3D space-time reality and overcome the gravity of illness.

Only spiritual freedom will perform the right actions and bring about healing miracles.

Find and identify the tiny membrane separating perfect health from quantum illness.

You must thirst after knowledge. Search within, and in the immediate and remote environment.

A Second Opinion

Sometimes holistic healing needs a second opinion from a medical professional. A new QO may consult their spouse or partner, a friend or a family member.

At this stage of the healing process the QO can seek a holistic, medical opinion and undertake some further medical diagnostic steps. It could be a consultation at a trusted GP practice or a visit of a specialist. A second opinion could also be provided by a trusted acupuncturist or a massage therapist.

A fresh review of your test results can be very useful in the process of healing. It can be a cardio check, the electrocardiogram (ECG), an assessment of your stress levels or a measure of heart rate variability. It may be a Doppler ultrasound of the heart, an x-ray of the chest, a computer tomographic scan of the troubling body part, or an MRI scan.

Sometimes, the seemingly solid opinions of medical experts need to be questioned and you should engage in a courteous dispute.

Simple laboratory blood or saliva tests can be done to determine your genetic profile and check your inflammation level. Sometimes an ordinary lab test can give a revolutionary insight into the cause and the nature of a disorder. Unbiased interpretations of test results and imaging are essential for the knowledgeable QO. And the QO needs to analyse and interpret the results of medical examinations carefully and accurately.

Getting a second medical opinion will significantly increase the probability of creating a dominant frequency in the unified field, for healing to occur. But this is only true if all involved observers act in unity towards the intended goal of healing. If the engaged Quantum Observers are distracted by financial considerations or if they apply their business/research models, it will produce contradictory messages and a zero response from the fabric of the Universe. It can even make the symptoms worse.

Singluarity

If you suffer quantum illness, all that you need can be summed up in a single word: singularity. Healing requires a clear, unified direction of holistic healing and not an optional mind set. This is the attitude of a stable QO, who cannot be easily distracted. The QO is able to filter out all misleading, irrelevant or false information.

Altogether, 10 to 15 people may be engaged in the healing process of one person and in restoring the body's functionality. The skilled QO will focus on the unlimited potential for healing, on quantum entanglement and the interactions of our quantum heart and quantum body placed in the immediate environment. The associated partners, the sQO must be knowledgeable persons and dedicated to holistic healing. They can read and interpret the symptoms and they can be supportive in choosing the right action or to finding a cure. The unified field of energy for the healing process will then grow exponentially to reach a critical level, and create a quantum leap in the singularity-based curative process.

The human body is a self-organizing system and it needs verbal, affirmative feedback for coding DNA. Positive healing impulses will awaken the perfect quantum genetic imprint and accelerate genuine regeneration, coming from your clever, all-knowing genes.

Quantum healing can be a joyful, deeply satisfying process. The application and practice of this newly acquired healing knowledge will empower the intelligent heart and the quantum body.

Bodily phenomena, both physical and biological, generate the flow of energized electrons and play an essential role in sustaining health and vitality.

The huge amount of data amount provided by visual feedback, the intense observation of the changing body and diagnostic procedures, are all inputs that can become intelligent information. This acquired knowledge about the heart functions and the insights into the healing process can in turn cause the relocation of harmful information back to the invisible fabric of the Universe.

The assertive actions of the QO can create a window for the newly configured data relevant for healing to re-enter. The QO will assemble trillions of sub-particles to guide them in the right direction. This focused intention will collapse the probability waves and re-establish good health.

The quantum heart is a continuous battlefield in the process of holistic healing. The visible forces of 3D space-time are trying to get exclusive hold of it. We need to establish a new and advanced position of the quantum heart connected to the fabric of the Universe.

Acupuncture as a Quantum Medical Intervention

The practice of holistic medicine and the modern approach of the medical physics need a thorough understanding of the interactions between a therapist and a patient in the process of healing. Some aspects of holistic medicine can be more likely found and experienced in acupuncture clinics, because this traditional practice is holistic by its nature.

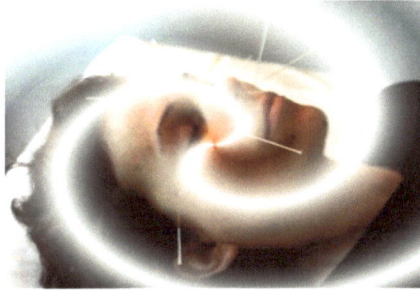

Figure 84 Acupuncture as a quantum medical intervention. The acupuncture needles interact with the human electromagnetic body field
Own work

Acupuncture is based on the central role of the heart, domesticating the spirit/shen. The heart, according to traditional Chinese medicine (TCM), acts as the emperor of the human body, shaping the expansion of consciousness. It follows that, if the heart is correctly understood by a skilled QO, the cooperation between heart and brain will become more intense, clear and coherent.

Acupuncture can reduce stress and bring relief from distressing symptoms, and restore the full functionality of the brain's default network DMN.

Recent work from the Chinese Peking University in cooperation with the Free University in Berlin performed by Yuqi Zhang at al. indicates that acupuncture positively influences the functionality of the default mode network. The study shows that, "increasing the 'dose' of acupuncture, by increasing the number of needles or the intensity of needle stimulation, might induce an enhanced modulation of DMN that persists even after the termination of acupuncture". Certain points on the scalp are acupuncture targets that improve the DMN.

The restoration of DMN is one of the targets of the practice of acupuncture.

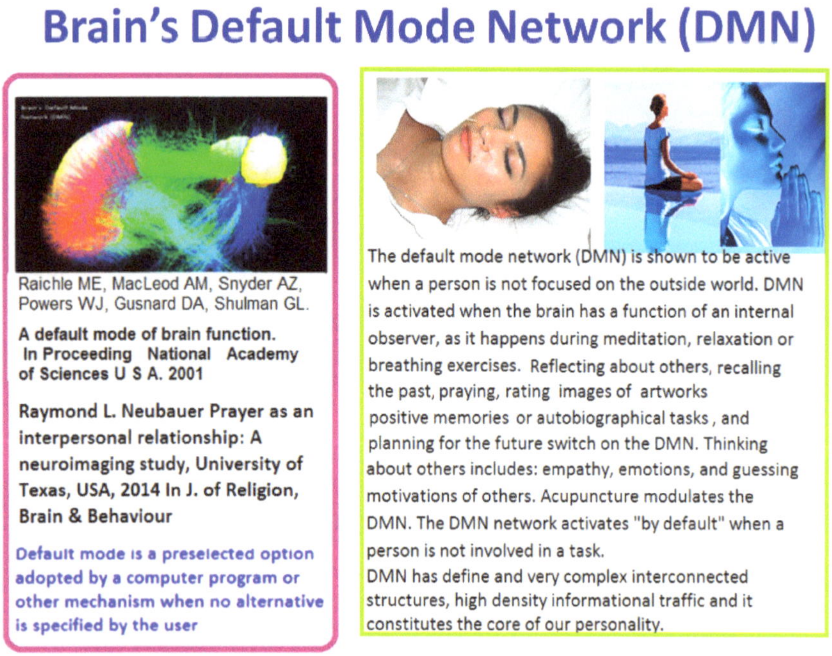

Brain's Default Mode Network (DMN)

Raichle ME, MacLeod AM, Snyder AZ, Powers WJ, Gusnard DA, Shulman GL.

A default mode of brain function. In Proceeding National Academy of Sciences U S A. 2001

Raymond L. Neubauer Prayer as an interpersonal relationship: A neuroimaging study, University of Texas, USA, 2014 In J. of Religion, Brain & Behaviour

Default mode is a preselected option adopted by a computer program or other mechanism when no alternative is specified by the user

The default mode network (DMN) is shown to be active when a person is not focused on the outside world. DMN is activated when the brain has a function of an internal observer, as it happens during meditation, relaxation or breathing exercises. Reflecting about others, recalling the past, praying, rating images of artworks positive memories or autobiographical tasks, and planning for the future switch on the DMN. Thinking about others includes: empathy, emotions, and guessing motivations of others. Acupuncture modulates the DMN. The DMN network activates "by default" when a person is not involved in a task.
DMN has define and very complex interconnected structures, high density informational traffic and it constitutes the core of our personality.

Figure 85 The brain default mode network is made up of defined anatomical structures in the brain. The DMN is a cluster of structures in the brain that keep the core of the individual personality active. These structures conduct very dense informational traffic because they hold and maintain the core of your personality
Own work with extract from Wiki Commons by Andreashorn DMN

The Electromagnetic Field

In order for there to be good connectivity between probability waves, your body needs to have a stable electromagnetic field.[http://www.abovetopsecret.com/forum/thread1004577/pg1.

The human body produces a stream of electrons forming an electrical current, and electric currents are always accompanied by electromagnetic field (EMF). The emission of bio-photons originating from the body creates movement within the EMF, forming electromagnetic waves. The quantum heart has a major effect on the body's field. It produces a strong bio-electromagnetic field. The body field has the power of 1/1,000 of the strength of the entire magnetic field of Earth. Put another way, the magnetic strength of a thousand intentionally united quantum hearts in human bodies is equivalent to the earth's entire magnetic field.

Increasing subatomic awareness is an important part of holistic healing. The human body is built from atoms and very small sub-particles vibrating at different frequencies. Every second of every day, your body interacts with billions of probability waves arising and collapsing within it. You must step through the door to the fabric of the Universe to meet the full potential for health.

Step through the door to the fabric of the Universe to meet the awaiting potential for health.

In his book *"The God Chord"* Robert L. Schrag speaks of the universe as a huge musical instrument built from very tiny vibrating superstrings. It constantly produces frequencies, sounds, tones and vibrations. The superstring theory describes the fundamental, irreducible building block of the universe to be the vibrations of superstrings. They play the intergalactic, universal music of life. Everything is built of these tiny superstrings.

Dr Schrag's work examines the implications of this cosmic music for the human heart. The book explores how universal, harmonic superstrings form the basis life, love and the fabric of the Universe. Many people perceive these weird, supernatural features of the fabric of the Universe as a sign and evidence for God's existence.

We humans are well connected to other quantum hearts via quantum entanglement. In fact, we are all interconnected. Everybody's growth, performance and maturity matters to everyone else, and the connections and their meaning unfold over the course of a lifetime. What you do affects all other living entities on Earth.

The Brain's Default Mode Network (DMN)

The default mode network in the human brain was first described in 2001 Raichle M.E. at al. It is made up of defined anatomical structures in the brain. The DMN is a cluster of structures in the brain that keep the core of the individual personality active. These structures conduct very dense informational traffic because they hold and maintain the core of your personality.

The major aspects of an individual's lifestyle are imprinted in the default mode network. And, importantly, quantum illness is coded in the DMN. This is especially so in the case of the double agenda, which originates in infancy and makes a powerful imprint in the core of personality.

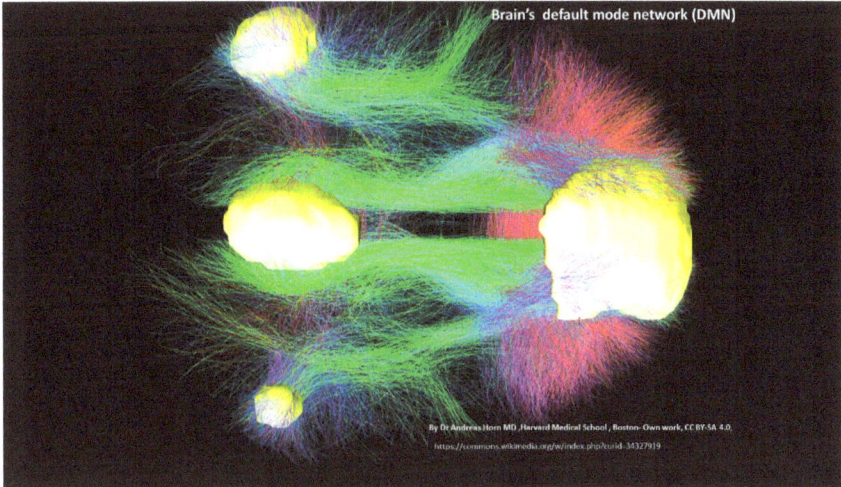

Figure 86 Brain's Default Mode Network DMN. The pathways
are dis-playing the informational traffic in the brain
Wikipedia Commons by Andreashorn

The DMN is always busy. As soon as you wake up in the morning the DMN uploads all personal data, recent events and information about the immediate environment.

The DMN is highly dependent on your oxygen and energy supply to function optimally. It can be strengthened by acupuncture, breathing techniques, meditation, prayer and positive emotions.

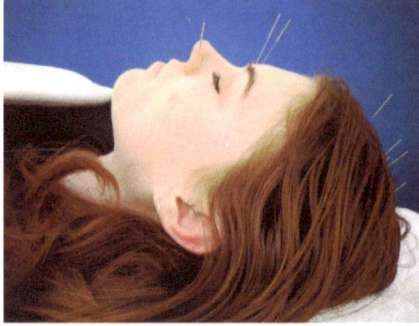

87. Acupuncture intervention to restore
the normal function of the brain's default
network DMN
Own work. Courtesy Joley H.

The restoration of DMN perfect functionality is one of the targets of the practice of acupuncture.

Optimal DMN functionality requires sufficient oxygenation and is linked to the intelligent functions of the heart. The loss of DMN functionality results in memory loss, total absence of vivid dreams and is seen in the end stage of dementia or in Alzheimer's disease.

Sometimes the informational traffic in the DMN is very dense, even chaotic. In Chinese culture, people use cold water or a cold pack application to cool down the extensive informational traffic in the brain's default network.

The electromagnetic function of the brain and the generation of electromagnetic waves can be displayed and measured as an electroencephalograph (EEG).

Quantitative ElectroEncephaloGram (qEEG) is a special kind of EEG where brain frequencies are coded and displayed as different colours. It allows reading the four particular frequencies in the brain more easily.

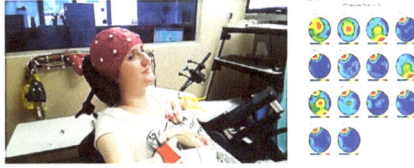

Figure 88 A patient undergoing qEEG.
On the right is the 4-colour display of the
EEG output
Own work. Courtesy Candice C.

Reversing the Double Agenda

When the personal self-reward system interacts with social or sexual taboos it is virtually untraceable. The traumatised person shows one face to their family and social environment, and a completely different face when pursuing personal and self-invented rewards. The success of a personal self-reward system lies in keeping it in secret. This is not difficult for the unlimited potential of a human. It develops a double agenda, which is the third component of a quantum illness. The double agenda changes the pre-designed trajectory of a natural and just flow of energy. It covers up the real information in 3D space-time reality. The double agenda bypasses 3D space-time reality and breaks into the untraceable virtual world of the mind and thoughts.

The 2018 film *"Molly's Game"* shows how quantum illness is interconnected with justice. The movie depicts all five stages of a quantum illness: the traumatized self, the personal self-reward system, the double agenda, the deal with death and the supertrauma. Molly can persevere and endure. Molly rages and offends her father in an attempt to get the desired reward, to win over the powerful man invading her private space.

In illness, the quantum heart loses access to the world of unlimited potentiality, to the intelligent information contained in the fabric of the Universe. It disconnects from the quantum reality of peace, health, harmony and truth. The fabric of the Universe is unforgiving if the affected person continues to make mistakes and tolerates the double agenda.

In the healing process there is no place for a double agenda scheme. To heal the traumatized self, the QO must assert an unwavering "Yes" to the healing practice and a determination to stop the double agenda and the self-satisfaction system.

Facing a disease can be a very dynamic, turbulent process. It challenges the quantum heart, the physical body and the DNA's intelligence. You can be in unchartered territory, facing unknown frontiers, which grow parallel to your gradually progressing spiritual development. No matter what burden appears, or whoever wants to hinder the healing process, it is essential to regain and hold fast to your autonomy.

There have been many breathtaking discoveries in the past 100 years. The chart shows major discoveries in quantum physics, quantum medicine, genetics, quantum biology and in the heart sciences.

100 Years of Major Discoveries

The timeline displays the magnificent progress of cardiology and the major discoveries in heart sciences, along with developments in modern genetics and molecular biology.

The major break-through discoveries have almost all been made in the last century. The scope of discoveries extend from the empirical revelation of traditional Chinese medicine (TCM), which more than 2000 years ago positioned the human heart as an emperor at the core of the human body, to the intelligent heart functions and its smart regulations. It includes the progress of medical physics and advanced computing with quantum computers which have been established in recent years.

Book 3: Healing the Embattled Heart

Here's what to do

1. Causes of Heart Attack and How to Prevent It

A premature, negative outcome for the human heart usually comes from overstimulation by stress hormones. The trigger might be one or more factors, such as:

- an adverse side effect of medications
- too many nutritional supplements
- recreational drugs
- insufficient oxygenation
- a low physical training level
- excessive consumption of coffee or alcohol
- long lasting exposure to work related or family stress
- a tragic event in the family or sudden loss of a loved one
- a financial or social crisis
- an accident.

Heart palpitations and chest pain often manifest prior to a heart attack or sudden cardiac death. An excess of stress hormones causes the down regulation of 7TM cellular receptors and the loss of cellular sensibility. Then a toxic trigger or an existing genetic predisposition can disrupt a precious life.

"The loss of cellular sensibility" means failing to recognise, or misinterpreting, cardiac warning signs. Our modern lifestyle exposes every individual to many harmful factors. And any such factor can be a forceful trigger for abnormal heart beats or coronary artery spasm. These risk factors develop a cumulative, negative load on the heart and can severely disrupt the heart's performance.

The disruption of the heart's normal function comes mostly from uncoordinated and incoherent heart/brain interactions, and from a poor energy imbalance. It could be a hormonal or mental imbalance producing a moment of confusion that in turn results in uncoordinated heart action. Then the human heart starts to fail and loses its beautiful precision and flexibility.

"Broken Heart Syndrome"

An imbalanced lifestyle can cause heart weakness. Particularly in the matter of women's health, the heart is at high risk due to its inherited and very different anatomy in comparison to a man's heart. The constitution of a female heart may not be strong enough to withstand the negative impacts of the traumas of modern life, and may express itself in exceptional circumstances known as a "broken heart". "Broken heart syndrome" is a medical condition discovered in Japan. It was called Takotsubo Cardiomyopathy because of the specific shape of the affected left chamber of the broken heart. In this condition he left ventricle of the heart is enlarged. It does not pump enough blood. When contrasted during a cardio procedure is very similar to the Takotsubo, a Japanese trap used to catch octopus. https://www.health.harvard.edu/heart-health/takotsubo-cardiomyopathy-broken-heart-syndrome

"Broken heart syndrome" feels like a heart attack with typical chest pain and dizziness. However the hallmark of a heart attack, a blockage or a spasm of the coronary artery, is missing. Medical research suggests that up to 5% of women evaluated for a heart attack actually have "broken heart syndrome". Broken heart syndrome often goes unrecognized.

Electrocardiogram (ECG) and Heart Rate Variability (HRV) tests are very useful tools in the evaluation of an individual's ability to cope with distress, and they aid in detecting stress related disorders. HRV testing is important in checking the intelligent heart functions.

The intelligent heart performs its enormous workload day and night, 24/7. It continuously and precisely adjusts the volume of ejected blood in time according to the demands of the body and rapidly occurring changes in our environment. The intelligence of your heart decides the timing of the contraction and the amount of blood to be ejected with every single heartbeat. It is extremely finely tuned. It needs a highly developed intelligence running multiple on-going calculations and adjustments due to the impact of the unpredictable influences caused by rapidly changing environment, mental impacts, fluctuating levels of stress hormones, and changes caused through alternating breathing patterns. These factors need to be assessed by your GP at every consultation.

The GP will typically ask some medical history-related questions and inquire about the actual symptoms. They will measure your systolic blood pressure (the first higher number, usually around 120) and diastolic blood pressure (during the relaxation of the heart, normally around 80 mm). They will check your heart rate (beats per minute) and sometimes check for abnormalities in the heart rhythm.

This standard examination may not discover elevated stress levels or hormonal imbalances. It may not indicate a deficit in the oxygenation of the body. It would need a more holistic assessment of the heart and the cardiovascular system in the form of a full heart check-up. This holistic, advanced examination will include an electrocardiogram and heart rate variability (HRV) measurements.

2. Prevention:
The Ten Foundations of Health

The heart has a holistic, supreme role in healing the whole body. The intelligent functions of the heart are an indicator of your existing connection to the electromagnetic field of the invisible fabric of the Universe.

The practical measurement of heart rate variability (HRV) and its visual feedback to the patient is an example how holistic medicine can be practiced. We can combine the data from an ECG chart with that of an HRV reading to produce a simple diagram that conveys the complexity of bodily states and processes to any individual. In this form HRV is an indicator of the capability of the QO to enable their cardiovascular system to reach its full potential. In a single image, we can see the internal balance and the functionality of the heart, and the respiratory and hormone systems.

The electromagnetic nature of the body is evident when we analyse its fundamental structures, present in every human cell. These cell structures include the intercellular connections: synapses and desmosomes, and the 7TM receptors.

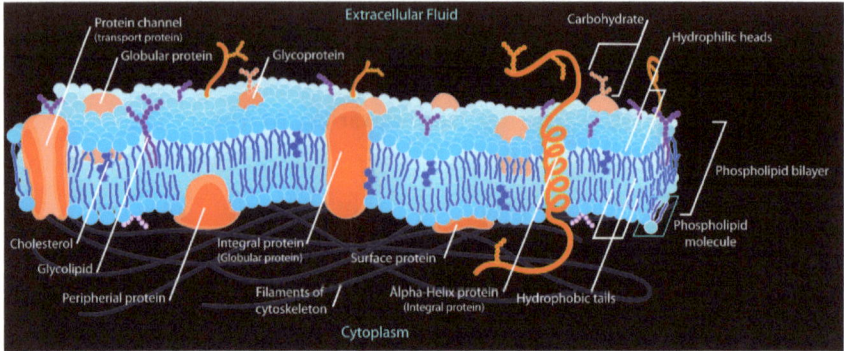

Figure 89 The cell membrane
Wikipedia Commons by LadyofHats Mariana Ruiz

Medical acupuncture is effective because it interacts with the electromagnetic components of the human body.

In his landmark 2009 study of acupuncture, *Prospective Tests on Biological Models of Acupuncture*[Department of Medicine, Cambridge Health Alliance, Harvard Medical School, Evidence Based Complementary Alternative Medicine, 2009, https://www.ncbi.nlm.nih.gov/pubmed/18955283. Dr Charles Shang from Harvard Medical School showed that the established acupuncture points on the skin surface have measurably higher electric conductivity, stronger electrical current and a high density of gap junctions.

Dr Bruce Lipton was the first scientist to observe an electromagnetic receptor in a cell. He described it as a dish or an antenna because this type of receptor detects not only bio-chemicals and hormones but also electromagnetic waves.

Electromagnetic receptor

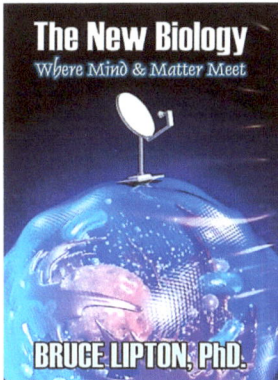

- The cutting edge research in molecular biology has ben done by Bruce Lipton in 2005
- It reveals that every cell of our body has a special receptor like an antenna, a dish sensing all kind of frequencies
- It can receive electromagnetic waves, acoustic frequencies, light and bio-photons

90 Electromagnetic receptor in Bruce Lipton's book "The New Biology
Own work with the image of the cover of the Bruce Lipton's book "New Biology"

He also discovered that the cells' brain is not the DNA in the nucleus but the membrane of the cell. The membrane of the cell separates the inside from external world. The membrane is highly selective for many substances regulating the intake of minerals, water and nutrients.

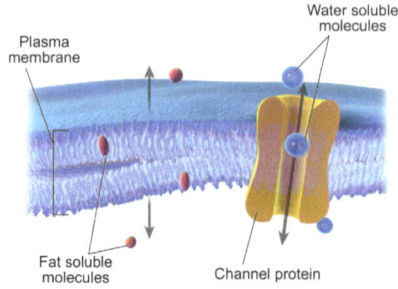

Diffusion Across the Plasma Membrane

Figure 91 Movement of water and water soluble substances through the cell membrane
Wikipedia Commons by Bruce Blau

The membrane creates electromagnetic potentials which allow the activation of muscles, including the heart muscle. It prevents toxic substances entering through its guarded gates. It has hundred thousands of receptors.

For these reasons Dr Lipton called the membrane a computer chip (the hardware) and the DNA is the program (the software), which can be overwritten. This is the power of epigenetics.

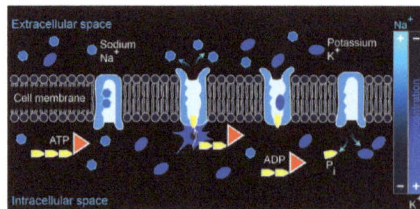

Figure 92 The cell membrane creating the electromagnetic potential trough movements of ions of Sodium and Potassium
Wikipedia Commons by LadyofHats Mariana Ruiz Villarreal

Now, in the age of Covid 19 vaccinations, the membrane is forced to produce the corona virus protein spikes. However, because of its intelligence the cell membrane cuts off the protein spikes (cleavage or sharp division, split), which can be a significant amount of the proteins able to promote the development of clots in the blood.

Signs and Symptoms

The main task of a QO is to build a core of knowledge about the functionality of the body and its monitoring. Some important indicators to monitor and follow up are:

- heartbeat
- pulse and pressure waves
- blood pressure (BP)
- diaphragmatic breathing

Diagnostic imaging procedures can be immensely helpful in delivering accurate information to the supervising mind of a QO and will provide the relevant diagnostic information.

Once the information is mapped in the mind it will be conducted to the coding DNA.

The first step is to identify unhealthy processes in the body and their origin, based on the signs and symptom. This process of examination and investigation is known in medical terms as the diagnosis. For example, you should take note of tension in muscles and tendons, especially in the shoulder area, as they are connected to the heart functions.

Simply watching the body's temperature can be important. By checking for cold hands and feet you'll have information about the effectiveness of blood circulation. Feet are the most distal (furthest from the heart) parts of the body and their undersupply can be the first sign of weakness in the heart.

Biofeedback

One of the basics of medical physics is understanding and awareness of the body's electromagnetic field. The intentional observation of the body comes about through visual confirmation (collecting data) and the assessment of the data. This is called bio-feedback, which is a combination of your own subjective experience and measurable data points. Bio-feedback can simply consist of regular measurements of your pulse rate during physical training, or it might be a computerized portrait of the heart with accompanying stress level measurements. This data enables you to calibrate the correct approach for therapeutic procedures, especially prior to and after an intervention. Such intervention could be acupuncture or a massage or yoga session, or an exercise program under a professional guidance.

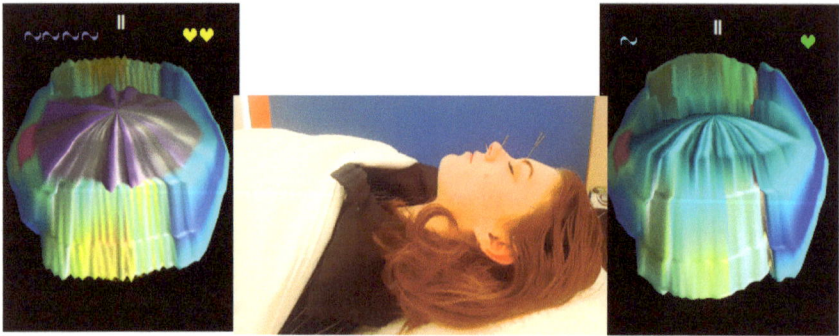

Figure 93 The picture displays two readings of a Cardio Image for the same patient before and after acupuncture. Note the positive change of the colours, the brown/violet coloration turned to blue/green, what is considered to be a sign of a significant reduction of the stress level
Own work

Biofeedback is just a matter of keeping an eye on things. You will accelerate healing and the maintenance of optimal health if you include as many non-invasive diagnostic measurements as possible in your daily routine:

- Pulse rate – at rest and during training,
- Heart rate variability,

- Stress index,
- Quantum resonance analysis,
- Blood pressure,
- Oxygen blood saturation,
- pH,
- Body weight.

And, where appropriate, get non-invasive visualisations, such as ultrasound, magnetic resonance imaging (MRI), etc....

Get into respiratory muscle training (RMT) so that appropriate breathing techniques become an integral part of who you are. Consider the intelligence of the heart at all levels of training. Monitor the extendable adaptability and plasticity of the brain.

The ultimate QO will combine knowledge originating from the full genome sequence, the metabolome, which represents the total number of important metabolites present within an organism, cell, or tissue, he/she would know a large scale DNA testing for the determination of the phenotype. QO appreciates the outer characteristics of the body, caused by epigenetics and will understand its practical applications. The knowledgeable QO will make the necessary changes in his/her lifestyle and will work to eliminate mental pollution.

Applied biofeedback is the primary tool used to re-pattern the breathing mechanism. The QO understands the plasticity of the human body and knows that regular oxygen dependent (aerobic) exercise, daily respiratory muscle training, intermittent fasting, and a healthy food will reshape the body in a short time.

Medical physics highlights an active and energetic water metabolism, the superconductors of the human body (silicon) and the ability to dope them with boron.

PROFESSIONAL QUANTUM OBSERVER pQO: A partner for the Quantum Observer QO

Holistic medicine compels us to find the right person, a medical professional or an allied health professional, to support us during the healing process. The pQO can listen and understand our health concerns. They could be a GP, an acupuncturist, a medical specialist, an exercise physiologist, a chiropractor, a dietician, music/play therapist, occupational therapist or a massage therapist. The common task of the teamed Quantum Observers will be creating a specific, strong frequency of healing to dominate the unified field of the fabric of the Universe.

The 10 Foundations of Healing

Here are the ten essential foundations of health, healing, and individual wellbeing.

1. Be a smart Quantum Observer
2. Oxygen
3. Water
4. Natural Light and Electromagnetic Waves
5. A second knowledgeable Quantum Observer (sQO)
6. Sound
7. Physical Exercise
8. Nutrition
9. Self-Medication and Prescription Drugs
10. Interconnectedness

1. Be a SMART Quantum Observer

You are, or can be, the Quantum Observer. As the QO, you'll use your brain and mind to map 3D space-time. The QO realizes the limitations of 3D space-time reality and deploys the intelligent heart and its operational tool, the spirit, to explore the invisible, electromagnetic dimensions of the fabric of the Universe. The correct exploration of this quantum reality produces a grid of consciousness (or 'spirituality' in the language of the 20th century) as an operational program. Using a quantum probabilistic approach, the QO observes and connects deeply with the functional body.

2. Oxygen

Efficient breathing and good oxygenation of the body is fundamental for intelligent heart functions, brain processing power and connection to the fabric of the Universe. Jesus Christ transferred the Holy Spirit to his disciples using the force of breath: *"Then he breathed on them and said receive the Holy* Spirit". https://biblehub.com/catholic/john/20-22.htm

These statements underline the importance of breath and oxygen for the optimal functioning of the intelligent heart and the stability of the electromagnetic field of the body. The use of abdominal, diaphragmatic breathing and daily respiratory muscle training are essential for optimal health.

3. Water

The quality of water we consume has a big impact on our health status. Water contributes significantly to the electromagnetic constitution of the human body. A water molecule contains two atoms of hydrogen and one atom of oxygen. Hydrogen is the simplest atom and is made up of just two particles: a proton and an electron. Protons are spinning continuously, giving the water molecules an electric charge, orientation and producing its magnetic field. The human body consists of 70% of water.

The electromagnetic constitution of the Human Body

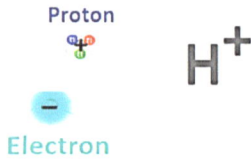

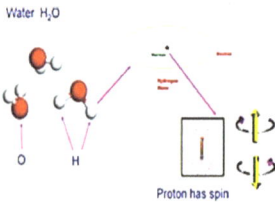

Proton

H^+

Electron

Water H_2O

O   H

Proton has spin

- Two hydrogen atoms are the part of a water molecule
- Every hydrogen proton has a spin and acts as a mini magnet in the Human Body
- Our body consists in 70% of water

Figure 94 Electromagnetic water in the human body
Own work

1 ml of water in the body contains more than 6 trillion hydrogen protons; a number that is hard to imagine. Here is what it looks like written out in numbers: 6,000,000,000,000,000,000,000. A single human body contains 252,000,000,000,000,000,000,000 of small spinning and charging magnets. Each of these tiny particles is part of the electronic matrix making up the body's electronic field, and directly affecting our health.

The electromagnetic constitution of the Human Body

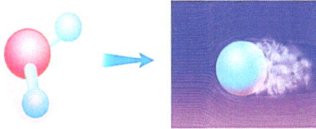

1 ml of water of the body contains more than 6 trillions of hydrogen protons, the number which is hardly to imagine
6,000,000,000,000,000,000,000,000
In 42 litters water in a body of 70 kg there is a vast number of
252,000,000,000,000,000,000,000,000
of small magnets

Figure 95 Electromagnetic constitution of the human body
Own work

The water we drink is also an important source of minerals such as Potassium, Magnesium and Sodium. These minerals support the smooth flow of electrical currents within the cell and tissues. Water cannot be substituted by any other drink.

In pursuit of good health, many of us have switched to drinking filtered water. Considering what's found in tap water these days that is an understandable approach. However water filters can go too far in the other direction, removing almost everything from our water, leaving it stripped of minerals altogether.

Drink alkalizing water such as Kangen water, which is standard tap water that has been changed according to quantum effects and is still rich in minerals in comparison to other water purifying systems. This will support the metabolism of minerals. Activated carbon as a filter is a part of the Kangan water process and this act to reduce the ingestion of plastic micro-particles.

4. Natural Light and Electromagnetic Waves

Our bodies need an abundance of natural light and adequate exposure to sunlight. The body is electromagnetic by nature and our cells interact daily with the electromagnetic waves generated by the sun. Our brains need the stimulating effect of daylight, transmitted through the eyes.

The brain is the most researched of all our internal organs and it is a model of how our organs respond to electromagnetic fields. But the heart generates the strongest biological electromagnetic field (EMF). And the heart's electromagnetic profile is very well researched because, during the millions of electrocardiograms performed around the world every day, every heartbeat is tracked. Scientists are studying how the entire body generates an electromagnetic field, and how the body's field interacts with external EMFs. Two scientific studies performed by Isakovic J. at al. in 2013 and 2018 focused on this, confirming the electromagnetic nature of the human body.

Great progress has been made in conventional and complementary medicine in identifying the electromagnetic functions of the heart and all the cells in our bodies as evident from the study made by Foletti A. at al.

Prospective Tests on Biological Models of Acupuncture
by Dr Charles Shang from the Harvard Medical School

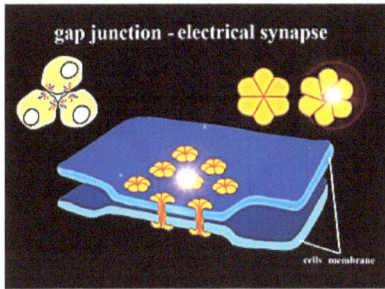

Acupuncture points (organizers) have high electric conductance, high current density and high density of gap junctions

https://en.wikipedia.org/wiki/Electrical_synapse

Dr Charles Shang: **Prospective Tests on Biological Models of Acupuncture**
Department of Medicine, Cambridge Health Alliance, Harvard Medical School, Evidence Based Complementary Alternative
Medicine, 2009, https://www.ncbi.nlm.nih.gov/pubmed/18955283

Figure 96 Electrical synapse in the human body
Wikipedia Commons by Mariana Ruiz LadyofHats - the diagram i made myself using the information on this websites as source: [1], [2], [3], and[4]. Made with Adobe Illustrator. Image renamed from File:Gap cell junction.svg, Public Domain, https://commons.wikimedia.org/w/index.php?curid=6027074

This prominent study cited above examined electrical and magnetic cell connections and their role during performing the medical acupuncture.

The human body consists of billions of cells, containing trillions of hydrogen proton-based nano-magnets, and an unaccountable number of connections between the cells that act as an electromagnetic switching network, receiving and decoding information and creating electromagnetic waves.

Our bodies also have an unaccountable number of electromagnetic cell receptors. These receptors were first time described by Dr Bruce Lipton in 2005 and compared to the satellite dish or an antenna.

In early 2000 Lipton was researching Parkinson's disease. He studied human cells using an electron microscope and found that every cell has a receptor that acts like an antenna as pictured as the image below. In fact the research following his ground-breaking discovery confirmed that every cell is equipped with hundred thousands of these receptors.

Exactly seven years later, in 2012 Dr Lipton's discovery was confirmed by Professor R. Lefkowitz and Dr B. Kobilka. They were awarded with a Nobel Prize in medicine/physiology for having mapped the 7 TransMembrane (7TM) receptor. They discovered how special proteins "G proteins" act as molecular switches inside cells and are involved in transmitting signals from a variety of stimuli outside a cell to its interior. They are coupled to 7TM receptors and conduct information to our DNA.

5.   A Second Knowledgeable Quantum Observer (sQO)

The journey to health, healing and wellbeing should not be undertaken alone. Enlist the help of a trusted person who can direct additional positive intentions to the healing process. Your sQO must be supportive and well versed in the probability approach to healing. The support of a sQO will help to collapse the probability waves which in turn will manifest the specific, required frequencies of the healing process. The presence of additional Quantum Observers will amplify the frequencies necessary for achieving optimal health.

6.   Sound

The sounds of daily life play a critical role in establishing and maintaining good health. Sounds are analogue frequencies, unlike radio and other electromagnetic frequencies, but sounds are no less important.

It's a good idea to do a sound audit. Identify the incessant sounds that add stress to your days. Pay attention to the sounds that pervade your life at home and at work. Just pause sometimes during the day. What can you hear? Air conditioner? Traffic? Kitchen noise? Chatter? Offensive background music? Whatever the sounds are that grate on your soul, do your best to eliminate them.

But also be sensitive to what is *missing*. While it is important to quell the harmful sounds around you, the active application of beneficial analogue frequencies is also important. Every day you should listen to music that pleases you and to the sounds of nature like the ocean or birdsong; and consciously practice singing or playing music,

7.   Physical Exercise

It is indisputable that regular, appropriate exercise is essential for health. But, whatever fitness system you deploy, you will always gain added benefits from breathing correctly during your routine. During exercise, focus your awareness on all your bodily functions and practice abdominal breathing. Apply abdominal breathing during walking, interval training, Pilates... Be aware of the value of respiratory muscle training during yoga, active meditation or any other physical activity. Correct breathing can activate your body's immune system, prevent viral or bacterial infection and reduce the stress. It can reinforce your connection with the fabric of the Universe and support its healing powers.

8.   Nutrition

A balanced, healthy nutrition is essential to maintain good health.

The nutrition is an integral part of a healthy life style. Traditionally food has been viewed as a source of energy, but we know now that food has profound interactions with our DNA affecting our wellness, well-being or even health. Every intake of food has an imprint on our DNA and has consequences at the molecular level for our bodily performance. Food components can turn on or off our genes altering the gene expression.

The progress in our understanding of genetics has opened new avenues to study interactions between nutrition, gene expression, genetic variability, health, and disease. The new discipline known as nutrigenomics considers the relationship between specific nutrients and gene expression.

Our genetic code is ancient. The modern processed food and nutritional daily habits can be on a collision course with our genetic make-up. So it is easy to understand that the cardiovascular diseases, heart attacks, immunological disorders, cancer and allergies are increasing.

The emerging evidence shows that the healthy nutrition should match the individual DNA. Individual nutrigenomics can help to prevent and even improve abnormal body conditions.

These are the eight individual and personal suggestions for healthy food choices:

1. We are designed as an unique system and it requires an individualized nutrition
2. We have genetically different taste preferences for different foods
3. We make a variety of nutritional experiences conditioning pleasant and unpleasant foods
4. In our genetics are also encoded the generational nutritional experiences
5. According to the contemporary research our habits in our daily lifestyle make an lasting imprint on our genes
6. We can have pre- programmed reactions to specific foods resulting sometimes in allergies
7. The food experiences in our childhood can determine our adult nutrition choices and can contribute to food intolerances
8. The local and seasonal food availability allows imprints on our genetics

There are some orientations and nutritional guidelines we have adapted to, and some of them we like or do not like. Nutrigenomics as a modern discipline can help us in the decisions for food choices. The acquired gene expression is above genetics and it is the most fundamental level of our health and bodily development.

The food choices have to include a variety of potent vegetables such as fennel, beetroot, sweet potatoes, cauliflower, yam and broccoli. Follow a nutrition that takes account of your individual genetic profile and unique metabolism. A nutrigenomic based plan combined with periods of fasting or reduced calorie intake will bring the desired results.

A complete the healthy 21st century diet, includes fresh pressed juices, preferably pineapple with lemon, carrots with ginger. The ultimate 21st century diet has also occasional fasting. There is no more effective detox than a simple fast. Fasting accelerates regeneration.

9. Self-Medication and Prescription Drugs

The careful application of natural self-medication: herbal teas, plants such as, *Artemisia vulgaris* (mugwort), *Artemisia absinthium* and sweet wormwood *Artemisia annua* can be supportive in the era of Coronavirus pandemic. As the scientific community searches for a cure for the Coronavirus it is good to recall and apply some of the wisdom of traditional medicine.

Contemporary research concerning the fight against the Covid19 virus focuses on chloroquine, a drug used for Malaria. https://www.news.com.au/lifestyle/health/health-problems/coronavirus-australia-queensland-researchers-find-cure-want-drug-trial/news-story/93e7656da0cff4fc4d2c5e51706accb5

The French researchers led by Phillippe Colson from the Aix-Marseille Université published in March 2020 an article entitled "Chloroquine for the 2019 novel coronavirus SARS-CoV-2" in the International Journal of Antimicrobial Agents.

Unfortunately Chloroquine, as a synthetic drug, has a long list of side effects. In particular, heart rhythm problems have been associated with higher doses of this anti-malaria agent. https://www.mayoclinic.org/drugs-supplements/chloroquine-oral-route/side-effects/drg-20062834

Herbal Adjuncts

The traditional approach to the anti-parasite and anti-malaria medicines includes the Artemisia plant family. These are very common plants that grow in nitrogenous soils, like weedy and uncultivated areas, such as roadsides.

The most two known of them are: Artemisia annua and Artemisia absinthium.

The Artemisia Annua research was awarded with a Nobel Prize Award in Medicine in 2015. https://www.nobelprize.org/uploads/2018/07/advanced-medicineprize2015.pdf

Aloe Vera, Horsetail tea and the application of Swedish bitters tincture on the skin (topical) or in small amounts of 3 to 5 ml internally can boost your immune system and support the function of your cardiovascular system and kidneys.

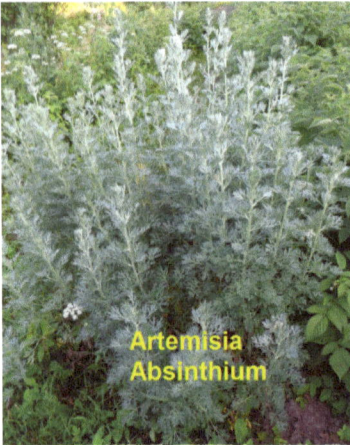

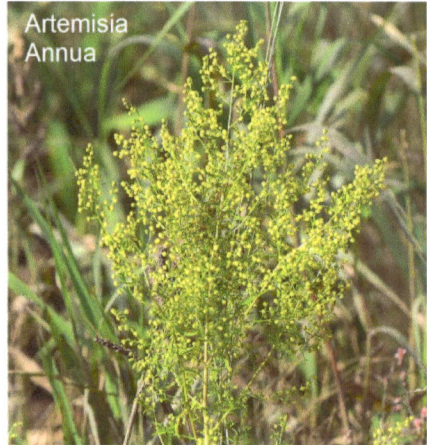

Figure 97 Artemisia Absinthium and Artemisia Annua.
Artemisia annua is known for its anti-malaria and anti-viral properties. Artemisia absinthium is known as a very useful agent against parasites, and it has anti-viral activity
Wikipedia Commons by AfroBrazilian, CC BY-SA 3.0 , via Wikimedia Commons

10. Interconnectedness

The holistic, intelligent human heart is interconnected with other people's hearts, from the first cellular appearance in mother's womb to the last breath and the final heartbeat.

You should embrace the interconnectedness of all humans and be aware of it. We are all interconnected at the level of quantum reality.

The advent of COVID-19 Coronavirus made the manifestation of this connection between people, tribes and nations noticeably clear. Our dependence on each other is now a serious matter of life and death. Applying the attitude of a QO and all-inclusiveness in a holistic view will support kindness and gentleness in complex human relationships. We are all humans and we are part of Planet Earth. We borrow the components for our quantum bodies from the earth. Spiritually we are one body in one spirit.

The process of reversing the heart's illness and regaining heart health requires the utmost attention and strong holistic awareness. Everybody wants to have a fully vital body. What is required is a structured, individualised heart health program, positive cardio experiences, a high degree of applicable cutting-edge cardio insights, and ongoing cardio training. Proactive cardio activities are the basis of successful positive heart remodelling.

Solid evidence that narrowed and blocked coronary arteries can be reversed was first shown by pioneer American cardiologist Dr Dean Ornish in 1999. He delivered scientific evidence that stenosis (narrowing) in the coronary system can be reduced by an individualised and holistic treatment approach. Dr Ornish is an acclaimed international speaker and the author of many medical books. He is also a health advisor to former US President Bill Clinton, who underwent bypass surgery some years ago.

Each of us can make the shift from a negative cardio situation to a good outcome by positively remodelling the heart and finding our way to a new, individual, holistic cardio lifestyle. This is the only way to master individual genetic disadvantages, to change gene expression and to upgrade down regulated 7TM.

G Proteins and 7TM Receptors

Above all, with a new, individualised cardio-oriented lifestyle it is possible to sideline or override the black imprints of one's genetic make-up, the generational, negative load of inherited junk DNA.

Recent discoveries about the role of 7TM receptors in cellular communication and the discovery of G proteins have opened the way to understanding how our heart acts and executes its superiority in your body.

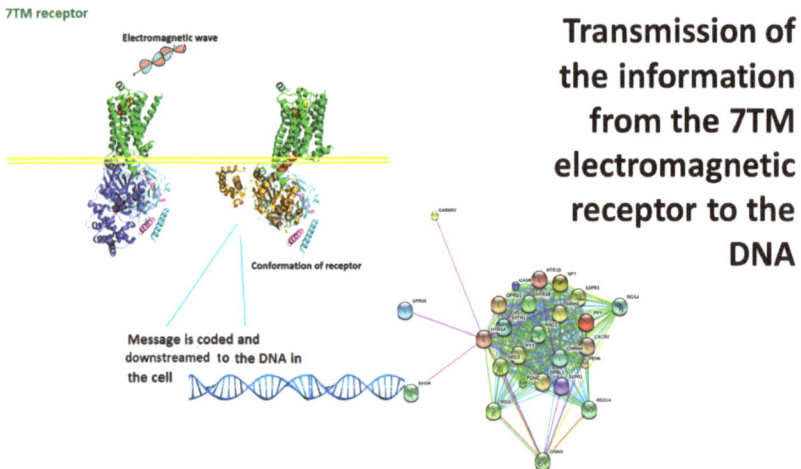

Figure 98 Transmission the message from the electromagnetic receptor to the DNA. The message is coded through the change of the shape of the receptor
Own work

G proteins are on the inside of the cell membrane (red colour). G proteins are internal messengers; they down-stream the impulses to the interior of the cell, to the nucleus, the dwelling place of our cellular DNA. The 7TM receptors are at the surface of every cell, its outer membrane. The G proteins are attached to every 7TM receptor. They are the sophisticated instruments of sensing, translating and down-streaming any information approaching our cells. 7TM receptors regulate many pathways including the cardio related stress cascade, sugar and fat metabolism, and the emotional responses of our heart. G proteins regulate the DNA responses to the impulses picked up by 7TM receptors. 7TM receptors and G proteins regulate the activity of the heart and circulatory system, the utilization of oxygen in the process of cellular breathing, energy management and optimal responses to energy crises.

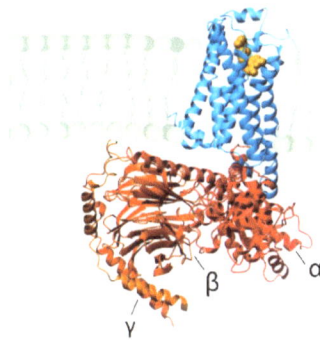

Figure 99 The crystalline structure of an activated 7TM receptor (blue colour) and its interaction with a hormone marked yellow (for example Adrenaline)
Picture adopted from the information for the public, Nobel Prize in Chemistry in 2012

3. Three Components of Individualised Heart Health

There is one thing that the QO needs to be sure of from the very beginning of the curative process: There is always an effective treatment for quantum illness.

A good way to start your journey to health is a breathing session or respiratory muscle training. You might use some natural medicines that are at home. Then consider holistic treatments like acupuncture, reflexology or remedial massage. This will calm unstable energy levels and bring instant relief of symptoms.

The first goal in the plan for quantum healing is to naturally relieve pain or other troubling symptoms. The second priority is to gain more energy.

These extended actions for healing will lead the receptive QO further and deeper into the territory of the second and third law of medical physics. More entangled QOs can create a stable, coherent and symmetric body field for healing.

As more specialised diagnostics are performed, the QO gains more knowledge and their strength increases. A team of engaged medical experts is essential to recovery: a technician who performs a procedure, a specialist who conducts a physical examination and reviews our results, the radiologist reading the scan or x-ray. They are very welcome Quantum Observers in the process of healing.

Sometimes, a simple natural agent such as a glass of fresh pressed pineapple juice mixed with lemon juice can be very helpful. It can very quickly terminate warning symptoms and temporarily restore the disturbed balance of health. Of course, we can't assume that all steps for healing will always be clear and precise. There are so many influences in the modern world. An individual is always exposed to many disturbing factors, distracting situations, and many forms of interference. That's why a comprehensive and holistic treatment plan is needed, and the QO has to be totally focused on this plan.

The Experienced Body

The enormous pace of new insights and the breakthrough discoveries of cutting-edge scientific research have been breathtaking. Recent advances in medical physics address three core directions for personalised medicine and a foundation for individualised heart health. Your holistic and intelligent heart builds an interface between:

1. Your inner space, within the quantum body
2. Your outer space, consisting of the direct environment in which you live (a home, a suburb, or a city)

3. The distant environment (the earth, stretching beyond the Karman line (at the height of 100 kilometres above earth) above all the way to billions of stars and a vast number of galaxies in space)

Your heart will exercise its interface via connections between the space above and the fabric of the Universe in a very smart way. It also reaches down to the tiniest particles and sub-particles. The heart takes control of many levels: electromagnetic, neuronal, hormonal, biomechanical, genetic, and much more. These three components: the human body standing and moving between outer space and the fabric of the Universe have an enormous impact on the life force of every individual and on the power contained in the genes. It creates an experienced and mature body. A holistic integration of these 3 components is needed in order to develop your awareness in 3D space-time. Integration is the engine of expanded consciousness.

By putting these principles into practice, everybody has the potential to re-shape, re-model and better understand the "experienced body", which is the vehicle for spiritual development. The experienced body is good looking, vital and energetic under any circumstances. It is stable and unshakable despite the strong impact of external weather conditions and worldly influences. The experienced body can overcome anything, even a strongest mental trauma; it can conquer a serious accident or a traumatizing injury.

The intelligent heart and the human body are acting to the rules of medical physics and both interact with the local and distant environment on the planet Earth. Your goal is to achieve the perfect orchestration of these three components: the heart, body and the dynamically changing environment. In summary:

1. The intelligent heart is your ultimate guide.
2. A well oxygenated body listens to its smart genes and heart, co-operating precisely with the brain in 3D space-time.

3. All-inclusiveness is based on inclusion of the local and global environment and at the same time the invisible nano-world of the fabric of the Universe.

In fact we are connected to these three components from the moment of conception. If you recognize that the human heart is a highly intelligent organ in action you will be well equipped to harness the subtle power behind coding and non-coding genes. If you reject the interactions of junk DNA you will become stronger, and more aware of your protective electromagnetic body field.

If you incorporate these insights into your experienced body, you will catch up with the 21st century standards of holistic heart health and better deal with the challenges of modern life.

The heart translates environmental influences and makes it comprehendible for all cells, tissues and internal organs, in a sophisticated process of a multilevel cellular communication.

4. Awareness of the Potential of the Human Heart

Achieving a state of full awareness in 3D space-time and knowledge of the hidden fabric of the Universe will accelerate the development of your consciousness. You will be able to build a mental image of the body, a new grid of graphical representation to map the invisible reality. This is the key to unleashing the heart's plasticity and its genomic potential for constant renewal. By pursuing the key genetic message of the heart (which is designed for 120 years of healthy functioning) you will extend your real lifespan.

The intelligence of the human heart has a very subtle, electromagnetic relationship with the human body. Your heart extends the body's living space about 1 metre around it, and its impact is far beyond the border of the body. Your electromagnetic body field can extend many metres, especially when you are in a supportive environment like the beach or countryside.

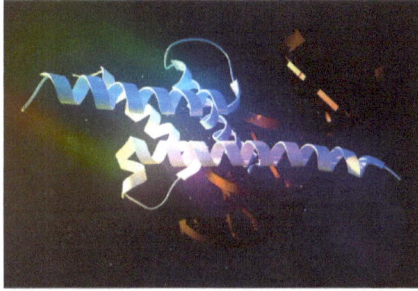

Figure 100 The CLOCK gene
Wikipedia Commons by Ismaïl Jarmouni

The synchronization of heart/brain interactions is governed by the CLOCK gene (Circadian Locomotors Outcome Cycles Kaput), which create an energy generating positive feedback loop.

The intelligence of the human heart can perceive critical information from the quantum world prior to the brain, and can sometimes predict future events.

A long lasting stress cascade will affect harmonious heart/brain co-operation and result in diminished energy production.

Perfect heart/brain cooperation relies on sufficient oxygen supply and water exchange between cells. Diaphragmatic breathing supports heart brain cooperation. A good supply of fresh, energized water will remove stagnant water from your cells. Air supply and water are two major factors in heart/brain cohesion and their harmonious team work.

5. *Individualised Heart Health*

The intelligent Human Heart has unlimited potential to maintain good health for the entire body, and to keep renewing itself for about 120 years. Recent discoveries about the sophisticated functionality of the human heart confirm the holistic design of our major internal organs and the heart's functional superiority.

Above all, medical research has provided a new understanding of the multiple, interconnected levels of the functioning of human heart. You need to integrate these new insights into your life. As a QO you can zoom down into body's cellular level, and receive a direct insight into the code of life, written in the genes. Then you will be able to make an impact on genetics and change your unique genetic expression. Once you have imprinted new, healthy habits in your daily life, epigenetics, the new genetic code itself will take the lead in your life, and you and your health will no longer be at the whim of the inherited genetic code.

Individualised heart health utilises modern science to integrate all these different aspects of health, and crystallises them into a cardio centred holistic approach. The individualised approach creates solutions for the negative loop of cardio related stress, which is dominating our lives in the 21st century.

6. Individualised, Holistic Health

Most heart disorders are preventable in a unique, individual way, but you need the right approach. And this involves you gaining a deep understanding of your heart and its functions.

The key role in healing is that of the smart Quantum Observer, who is deeply aware of:

- The unlimited potentiality for health of the fabric of the Universe according to the laws of medical physics
- The curative intention in the healing process; the realization that a QO can change the 3D reality of illness
- The crucial role of diaphragmatic breathing and of sufficient oxygen supply
- The practical application of bio-feedback and an understanding of heart rate variability (HRV) in diagnostics and healing

- The importance of cellular communication based on electromagnetic information processing
- The multiple levels of water functionality in the body, especially as an information carrier
- The great value of profiling DNA to guide the journey to individual health, please compare the study made by Johnson D. at al.

The knowledgeable QO needs to comprehend the importance of physical exercise in enhancing the ability of the heart to produce adult omnipotent stem cells and in counteracting the cardio stress cascade. All of this requires a reasonable level of determination from you, to put these insights into practice.

7. Becoming a Quantum Observer

The image below was created by my patient, Tony, a professional photographer. Tony made a very successful transformation after his heart attack and embraced holistic and individualised heart health. He discovered the intelligence of his heart and has put this knowledge into practice. Now, being a QO, he is taking the next step and progressing towards quantum heart knowledge, positively remodelling his intelligent heart and healthy body.

Downgraded receptors can be hidden, internalized or pulled in. Sometimes the receptors are not only trans-located into the interior of the cell, they can even be destroyed with a long lasting cardio related stress cascade, as it is displayed at the right side of the picture, where one 7TM receptor is missing in comparison to the left image.

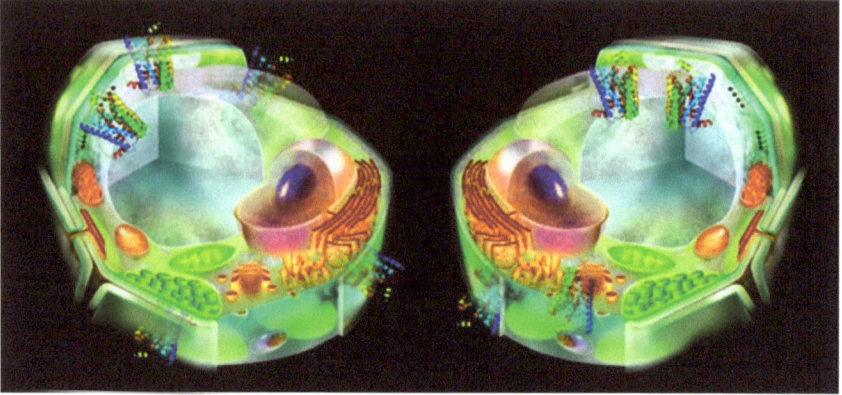

Figure 101 Downgrading of 7TM receptors
Courtesy Tony P.

In the picture, the left, normal sensing cell has 5 receptors (to simplify the image the number of 5 receptors was chosen, in fact in every cell are thousands of such receptors). Four of them (80%) are correctly placed at the surface and sensing all incoming impulses. In the right side of the picture, the receptors of the cell have been downgraded. Three of them are pulled (trans-located) into the cell's interior, one receptor is already missing, symbolizing a damaged or destroyed 7TM receptor.

It is more important now than ever before to be a knowledgeable QO, to prevent heart dysfunction, to stop an imminent heart attack or to conquer premature cardiac death. In the 21stcentury, not even one life should be lost because of lack of knowledge.

The smart QO must observe the heart and its intelligent messages and reactions. He/she needs to be sensitized to its subtle language. It is important to know the feeling of chest integrity, to recognize regular or disturbed heart rhythm, which sometimes feels as a missing heartbeat. This knowledge is necessary in order to correctly localize tensions, tightness in the middle of chest and to recognise that it is indeed originating from the heart.

It is very interesting that left hand first starts to ache by approaching dysfunction of the heart, by the heart palpitations, by angina pectoris or by heart attack.

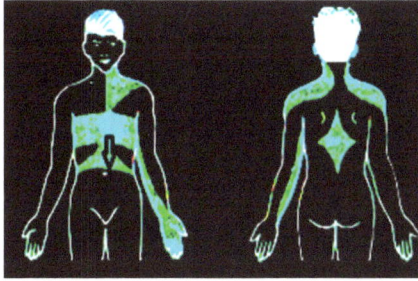

Figure 102 The common localisation of heartaches
Own work

The pictures above show on the left side the localisation of the typical pain caused by angina pectoris (tightness or burning feeling in the chest) or an approaching heart attack. On the right side the course of the heart meridian as it is displayed in the most books of acupuncture and traditional Chinese medicine. The direction of the spreading of the heartache and the course of the heart meridian match each other

Very often heart ache **slides down** to the stomach as is displayed in the picture. More than 90% of these strange sensations can be classified as symptoms of the heart. If you perceive any of the above symptoms it is time to take action.

It is not heartburn related to hyperacidity of the stomach. Heartburn originating from the stomach causes regurgitation of stomach acid and symptoms of indigestion. Heartburn from the digestive system is a burning pain or discomfort that **moves up** from the stomach to the middle of our abdomen and to the throat.

Awareness concerning heartache and its locations has to be newly mapped in the 3D space-time reality of your mind and in the awareness.

You need a focused sensitivity to any occasional numbness of your little fingers, to electrical pain in the jaw or to a burning feeling behind breast-bone. All of these symptoms are the warning signs of heart dysfunction.

A deeper understanding of heart science and more skills in deci-phering the coded language of the intelligent heart will provide more security and safety in dealing with heart symptoms. You must not fol-low confused, unqualified teachers and should not adopt, even uncon-sciously, the anti-life program of our generational junk DNA.

The knowledgeable QO will neither listen to messages of suicidal or lethal propaganda nor to the toxic digital codes of artificial intelli-gence. You will not follow the reactive impulses coming from the flesh, inherited from your ancestors' junk DNA. In fact these algorithms orig-inate from already dead people even if they want to be alive in the cho-sen body through inherited junk DNA, they would not get hold of the knowledgeable Quantum Observer.

This distinguishing wisdom is the key, the game-changer in the heart-killing mind-set based on a mechanistic view of the heart. To be successful in health creation, you must leave generational junk DNA be-hind.

QO needs someone at his/her side, with knowledge somebody who is friendly and really alive, who has already developed their own con-sciousness and mapped their new awareness. QO has to find someone who is already acquainted with the intelligence of his /her heart, and who knows how to listen and how to decode the language of the intelli-gent heart.

Warning Signs

A warning originating from the heart is usually a short event, lasting only a few seconds. It is a very significant experience but an inexperi-enced QO has no memory of it. All these are early warning signs sent by a troubled heart, indicating an increased risk of a Cardio incident:

- an occasional heaviness in the upper limbs

- pale face or deep blue coloured face with stagnated blood
- tiredness
- confusion
- momentary disorientation
- low or high blood pressure
- shortness of breath (SOB)
- agitation
- excessive sweating
- light-headedness with a tendency to faint.

If you experience one of these symptoms, take the right step and make a correct decision. There are no more than 10 seconds for the right decision: make a healthy DEAL with the intelligent heart to use the advanced and cumulative benefits of:

Diaphragmatic breathing

Exercises for respiratory system

Advanced cardio knowledge

Listening to the heart

Once the warning symptoms have stopped, you should perform a gentle breathing technique, yoga exercises or qigong — a traditional ancient training method to improve the circulation of blood and oxygenation of the body.

In the course of follow up, a visit by your trusted general practitioner GP, an individual genetic profile, genetically oriented balanced diet, and the use of proven natural therapeutic techniques can be considered: medical acupuncture, professional remedial massage, ear, foot, hand, and face reflexology.

Additionally an ECG, a Cardio check or stress test should be performed before any cardio high intensity interval training (HIIT) can commence, according to Dr Michael Mosley.

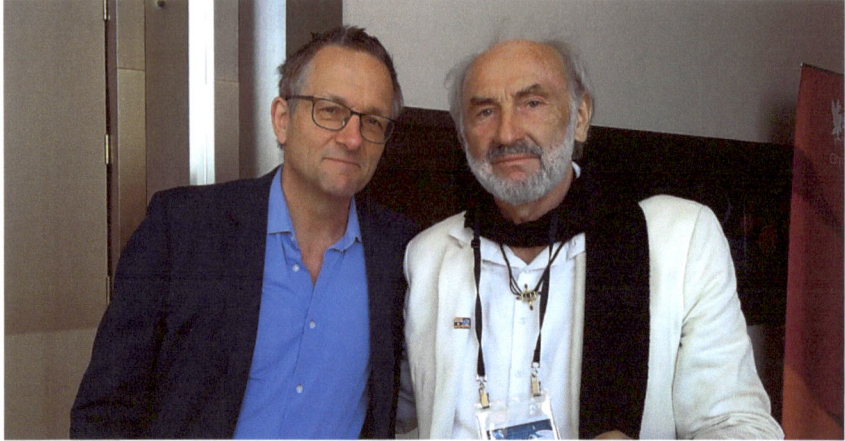

Figure 103 The author with Dr Mosley in Perth, Western
Australia during a medical conference Science on The Swan
in 2019
Own work

The unique, holistic heart is positioned at the centre of unlimited potentiality, the exciting territory of holistic health for the body, soul, mind and spirit. The advanced humans of the 21st century need to walk, to run, to dive, and to fly high, to go an extra mile in all of those areas, and to have joy with the perfect functioning of the intelligent heart, to encounter the majesty of life and the forces of health creation.
Symptoms-oriented training with 2 minutes of maximal, individually adjusted load, twice or three times a week can be beneficial to build a healthier lifestyle.

As a knowledgeable QO, you have a genius potential at your disposal. You can learn how to deal successfully with surrounding electromagnetic fields of the inner and outer space of man. You can be enthusiastic and can progress day by day to a bright future, supported by the power of the intelligent heart.

We must say NO to out-dated, simplistic, mechanistic, illness-oriented schemes and YES to individualised, holistic heart health intelligent directions.

Individual visions, missions, and plans will work out well when a QO takes the intelligence of the heart and the experienced body seriously. In order to be successful, your relationship with the intelligent heart needs to be built.

We strive to get better houses and cars, to build wealth, manage demanding jobs and become involved in local communities. All these need to be done to provide new and exciting opportunities for future generations. The expanding scope of communication, discerning fake news and readiness for 24/7 worldwide communication has to be mastered.

Our biological age can be reversed day by day as new awareness grows. The absolute challenge is not to be trapped by the time limitations of the best man-made clock. This is part of the new and accelerating challenge for health.

A total orientation towards the future is more important than ever before. The QO cannot be caught in the past, pondering the good old stuff and evoking the magnificent past experiences. It would be a backward-oriented mind trip. Journeying into the past is contrary to the future contained in the unlimited fabric of the Universe, the vibrating quantum holistic living matrix accessible by the intelligent heart.

If you are interested in the functional advancement of the human heart you must cross frontiers and reach out to the unknown territory of the holistic, intelligent human Heart. Continuous progress will expand your awareness and consciousness. This process needs strong dedication and an unshakable perseverance. It is a unidirectional process.

Your accumulated knowledge will build to a critical mass and then explode in spectacular insights.

Your personal development will jump to the next level in such a quantum leap as you've never experienced before. This is a journey with no points of return, because the way back, against the new awareness and consciousness, can bring destruction.

Importance of Knowledge about the Heart

A one way ticket on this exciting pathway will create exponential growth for you and those you love. It will produce a new quality of life. This will be a moment of great celebration. Feel it and be united at all 5 levels: heart, mind, soul, spirit and body. You are about to experience the incredible power reinforcing the inherent, immeasurable intelligence of the heart. This journey will produce never-ending wisdom of heart that works night and day in the inner and outer space of man, for the health and wellness of the individual.

The QO's Journey to the Nano Level

Your newly acquired knowledge can zoom you down, in your imagination, to the microscopic level and beyond. One step down from the surface of the body, close your eyes and enter the inside of your chest and see the heart as an intelligent and vital organ.

Descending deeper, contact and touch the molecular level. This is an amazing scene.

This view will reveal a fascinating, unfolding, nano picture of distressed cells losing their 7TM receptors (their utmost important sensors) and hiding their antennas. The cells are in distress, due to informational overload. You can see increasing pollution with micro particles of plastic and enormously toxic influences producing internal combat. The cells are fighting for survival and waiting for your focused, health creating intentionality of the smart QO.

Cardiac Sensibility

A temporary loss of the cells' internal sensibility not only limits the body's capabilities, it also narrows the horizons of an individual. The limited scope of our 3D reality awareness and our powerlessness in exploring the electromagnetic dimensions make us susceptible to many risks of daily life. This narrowed perception can cause you to react insensitively to those you love. This reduced sensibility and low sensitivity towards the external world can cause an accident or serious injury. The solution is to pay more attention to the body perception, its warning signs and symptoms.

The significant loss of cells' sensitivity can contribute to a catastrophic break down in health and can give rise to premature death in the form of the sudden cardiac death (SCD). Stable DNA and a trusted, experienced body are the tools you need to enhance the scope of your perception of the invisible aspects, and open the channels to the future.

Focus on the Intelligent Heart

In a state of perfect health everybody will take ownership of space beyond the earth. This awareness extends our reality without the need for GPS systems or other mobile apps. We need to focus on the intelligent heart to operate in a safe, superior mind mode. Expanded perception will accelerate the fusion of your awareness of 3D reality, the consciousness operating in the electromagnetic dimension of the fabric of the Universe and the outer space of man.

Nano-Satellites

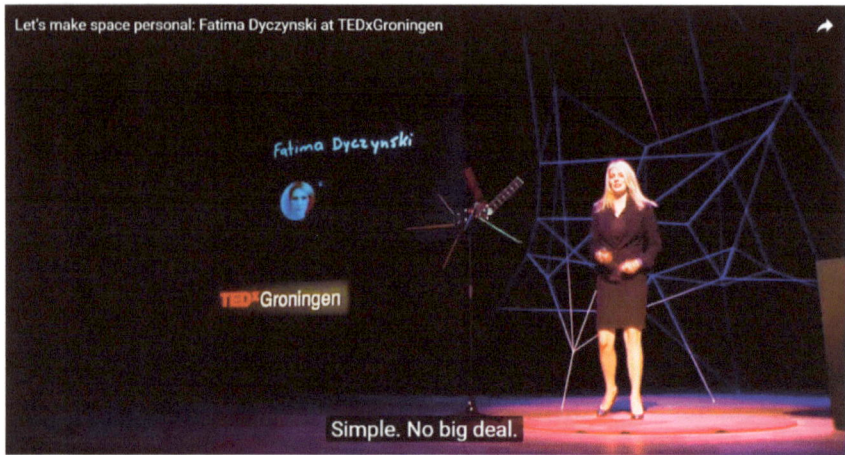

104. Daughter of the author Miss Fatima Dyczynski B.Sc.,
Aerospace Engineer during her TEDX lecture in The
Netherlands in 2013: "Make space personal"
*TEDx The Netherlands https://www.youtube.com/
watch?v=CJ0WhWLXsIE*

Most of us can already observe the weather forecast sent to our smart phones from a satellite. We can even virtually climb Mount Everest. In time, everybody will be connected to a personal nano-satellite. https://www.youtube.com/watch?v=CJ0WhWLXsIE

Your mobile phone will download an integrated bio-sensor with the necessary data for augmented reality, for perfect health and intellectual wellness.

Loss of Cardiac Sensibility and the Ignorance of Heart Science

The intelligent heart brings you closer to your holistic potential for perfect health. It supports your divine assignments and it will fulfil your life. It contains an ocean of knowledge which cannot be underestimated. Ignorance of the heart's communication will result in irregular heartbeats, palpitations and even heartaches.

No matter where you are positioned around the globe, you can experience the increased speed of negative reciprocity which can hit the heart like a boomerang.

Statistically, more and more cardiac deaths are predicted and the major reason is our loss of cardio sensibility. Billions of dollars have been spent on research to combat heart disorders and tremendous breakthroughs in diagnostic and surgical techniques have already been achieved.

What is needed now is an update of the mechanistic model of the heart and body.

The cause/effect mechanistic dogma in medicine and in the arena of holistic healing is next to useless in dealing with the heart's supreme dynamic position and its intelligence. Heart attack and stroke account for far more fatalities in our modern world than any other cause of death. Freedom from severe heart problems has still not been achieved, despite the rapid expansion of knowledge in medical science and sky rocketing technological advancement. The situation is very complex and we need an effective, dynamic, proven and individually-tailored medical care model to reach our ultimate potential. We are all predestined to discover the unique life force of the intelligent heart and the human body with its great plasticity and potential for positive remodelling.

QO Self Examination

The QO needs to be well skilled to quickly recognize an instance of instability in heart/brain communication and the missing coherence. Check your breathing mechanism several times a day, mapping it in your new 3D reality awareness. Zoom down in your imagination to the heart/brain cellular level and you can identify the early stage of negative, changed heart functionality.

You must quickly recognize any external interference, such as an external invasion of the electromagnetic field of the heart. If the QO is smart enough he/she can assess things and distinguish external and internal influences from each other. It needs to be done within 10 seconds.

8. Acupuncture

An acupuncture needle inserted in living tissue is a strong impulse for the self-organizing system of the human body. It a healing signal atcing at multiple levels.

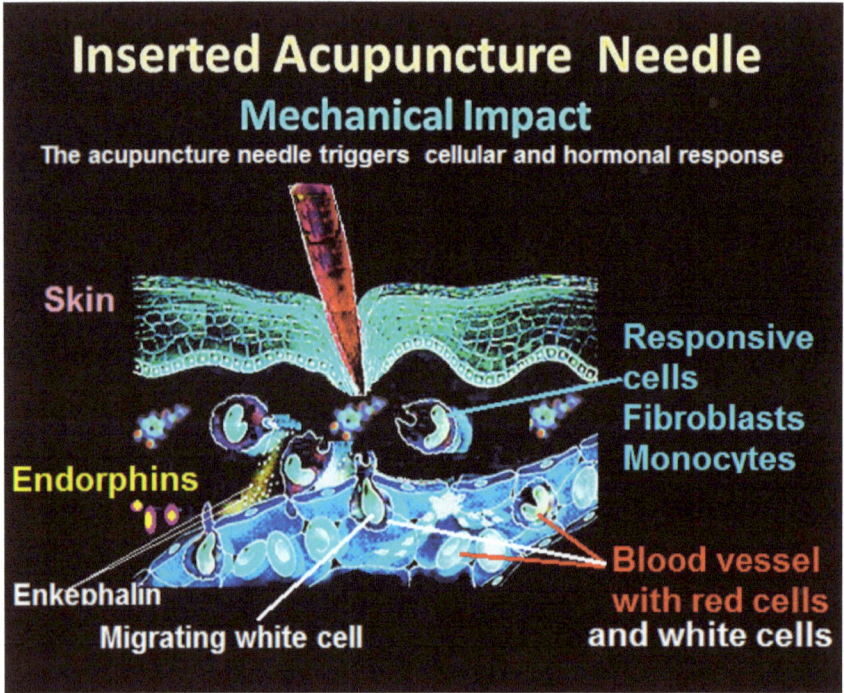

Figure 106 Acupuncture mechanical impact of the needle creates hormonal and cellular responses
Own work

The acupuncture point is a special area with a dense network of blood vessels, and receptors that regulate bodily functionality. It is also part of a bigger network of meridians crossing the human body and impacting the functionality of the internal organs.

The classic acupuncture needle is a strong mechanical impact to the tissue triggering a correct response.

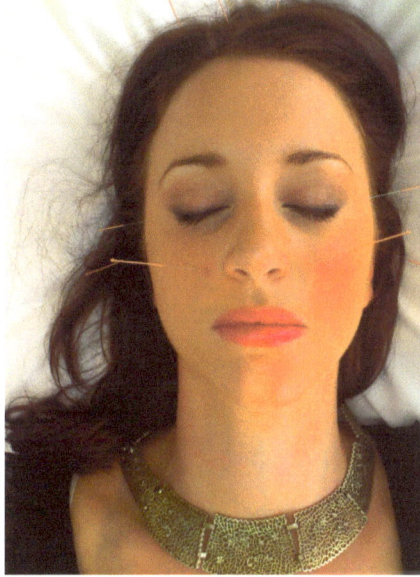

Figure 105 Classical acupuncture with
cooper handled needles
Own work

The classic acupuncture uses metal needles inserted into the acupuncture points to interacts mechanically and electromagnetic with the specific components of the body.

The needle creates a mechanical impact, triggers many cellular as well as hormonal responses and, as a pulsating piece of metal in the rhythm of the heart and the pulse wave, it modulates the body's electromagnetic field. After the needle is inserted the tissue releases β-Endorphins, the main hormones that stimulate positive mood and many other substances that help to regenerate the omnipotent stem cells and to accelerate the healing process.

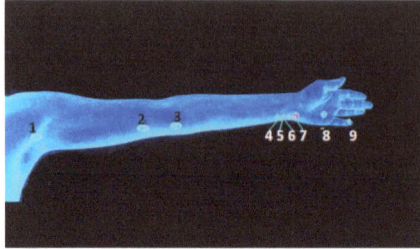

107 Heart meridian with all 9
acupuncture points. The seventh
acupuncture point H7 is known in
Chinese language as shenmen. It
means, translated to English, "the gate
to the spirit"
Own work

The classic acupuncture is used to treat functional heart disorders. The heart meridian then travels down from the arm pit to the inside of the forearm. It ends at the inside of the top of the small finger. The heart meridian contains 9 acupuncture points.

It is very interesting that left hand first starts to ache by approaching dysfunction of the heart, by the heart palpitations, by angina pectoris or by heart attack.

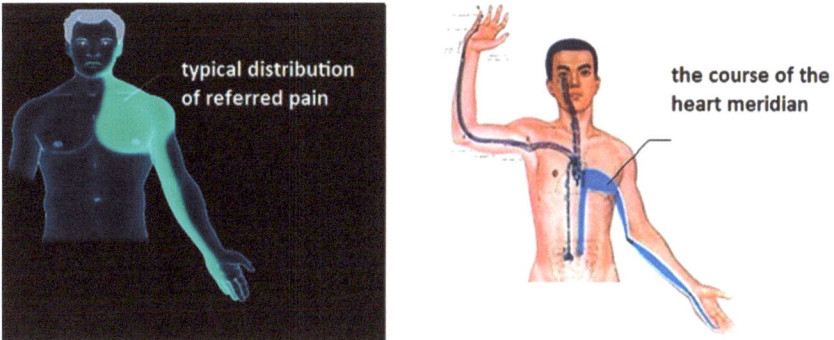

Figure 108 The image displays the localisation of the typical pain caused by angina pectoris (tightness of the chest) or a heart attack. On the right side the course of the heart meridian as it is displayed in the most books of acupuncture and traditional Chinese medicine
Own work

The direction of the spreading of the heartache and the course of the heart meridian match each other. One of the most important acupuncture points of the heart meridian is the point H7 known in Chinese language as shenmen. It means, translated to English, "the gate to the spirit". It is used to treat functional heart disorder and insomnia.

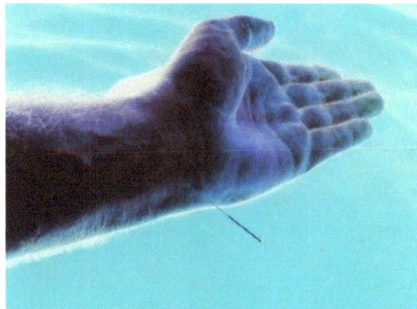

Figure 109 The acupuncture on the seventh point of the heart meridian H7, shenmen
Own work

The modern acupuncture forms such as electroacupuncture using the electrical impulses to stimulate the acupuncture points or magnetic acupuncture using a small magnets to influence the acupuncture points are also effective in the influencing the electromagnetic body. The ultra-modern laser acupuncture is also harnessing the influence of coherent light on the electromagnetic components of the body.

Even acupuncture without needles know as thermic acupuncture using the high temperature to stimulate the acupuncture points is effective because of the electromagnetic components of the human body.

Inserted needles causes localised bodily responses, but they also have far reaching influence, even on the brain's default network and the electromagnetic, morphogenetic field of the body. Medical acupuncture has a multidimensional framework of interactions with the human body. The response of the tissues to the solid metallic acupuncture needle occurs according to the laws of medical physics.

Acupuncture acts on The Electromagnetic Body

Acupuncture is also a quantum medical intervention. The water in the human body has an electromagnetic aspect. At the molecular level the body's most important electromagnetic components are hydrogen atoms. The hydrogen atom is built from a positively charged proton and a negatively charged electron. Hydrogen is a fundamental component of water and accounts for 70% of the body's weight. The electromagnetic features of the water contained in the body result from hydrogen's proton spin. The spinning protons in hydrogen impose an electric charge on the molecule, creating an electromagnetic field, so it acts like a tiny nano-magnet.

It is these vast numbers of the spinning hydrogen nano-magnets that are detected by MRI scans when they create an internal image of a body. The MRI scanner applies a strong external electromagnetic field and is able to bring a specific order to the random electromagnetically directed protons. Our internal organs all have different water content and so they show up as discrete objects in an MRI scan and they can be discerned from each other. Every tissue in the human body has a specific content

| 242 |

of water and this makes the difference in response to the external electromagnetic frequency as the magnetic field of MRI.

The cells of the human body are interconnected through specific electromagnetic structures, or "gap junctions", allowing their direct communication and information exchange. In a very real sense, bodily communication is based on a kind of a smart Wi-Fi network. Gap junctions are specialized connections between human cells, directly connecting the interior of the cells with the bio-plasma (cytoplasm) of the cells. Gap junctions conduct electromagnetic waves and allow electrically charged molecules to pass directly through these gates between cells.

An inserted acupuncture needle is a gentle electromagnetic message for the 7TM receptors and the G coupled proteins. The needle temperature is about 20 degrees Celsius in comparison to the body's 37 degrees. The temperature gradient causes a flow of electrons known as a weak electrical current.

This is a smart electromagnetic stimulation that is picked up by cellular receptors and connectors.

The Acupuncture Needle
Electromagnetic Impact

Temperature difference between human body and acupuncture needle of 12 Celsius degree create a gentle electrical current and an electromagnetic field

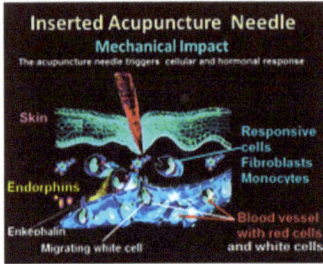

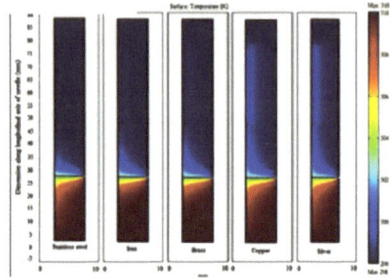

Tzou CH, Yang TY, Chung YC. Evaluation of heat transfer in acupuncture needles: convection and conduction approaches. J Acupunct Meridian Stud. 2015 Apr;8(2):77-82. doi: 10.1016/j.jams.2014.07.001. Epub 2014 Jul 22. PMID: 25952124

110 Acupuncture as a quantum medical intervention
Own work with an image from Tzou CH, Yang TY, Chung YC. Evaluation of heat transfer in acupuncture needles: convection and conduction approaches

Other fundamental building blocks of the human conglomeration of cells are the electrical synapse and the desmosome, the binding body. Desmosomes act like glue in binding cells together, sticking cells to other structures, and even holding the cell itself together. They determine the mechanical resilience of cell tissue and play an important role in intercellular communication.

An unhealthy increase of the intercellular communication can be a cause of headaches, unnatural sounds in the ears known as tinnitus and an increased stress for the cardiovascular system.

Headache - acupuncture treatment

Just after insertion of the acupuncture needles

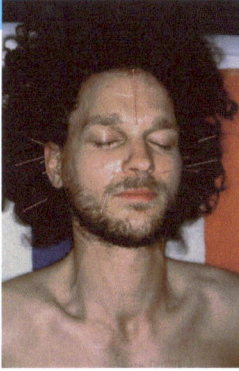

After 30 minutes of medical acupuncture

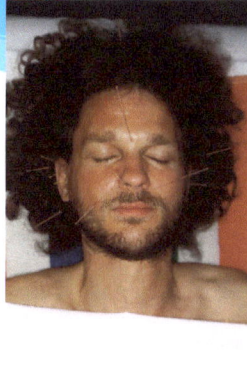

A 37 years old policeman was released from his chronic headache after three medical acupuncture treatments. Please note the increase of blood supply in the skin, deep relaxation of muscles, especially the shoulder region and even more electrified hairs

Figure 111 The image displays a 37 year old police officer who was released from his chronic headache after just three medical acupuncture treatment.
Own work

The prescription for headache, tinnitus and stress reduction can include following acupuncture points: Heart 7 Shenmen -H7, Pericardium 6- PC6, Lung 7- L7, Lung 9- L9-Taiyuan- influential point of vessels, Stomach 36- St36, Gall Bladder - GB34, Gall Bladder 43- GB43-Xiaxi, Kidney 3 K3-Taixi , Triple Energizer 5- TE5 Weiquan on the body and on the acupuncture on the head as displayed at the image: Governor Vessel 20- GV20 , Governor Vessel 26- GV26 Triple Energiser 17, TE17-Yifeng, Taiyang- Extra pont meaning in English "sun", Yintang – acupuncture Extrapoint meaning in English "moon", Gall Bladder 2- GB2-Tinghui, Triple Energizer 3-Zhongdu TE3 , GB20-Fenchi, and ear acupuncture.

Metabolic Independence

The intelligent heart can resist the suppressive forces of a cardiovascular stress cascade, a devastating mental distress, extreme weather conditions or long lasting, exhausting bodily workout. In these exceptional situations the heart recycles the stress mediators and releases active small molecules known as nitric oxide (NO). The abundance of NO in the circulating blood keeps the coronary vessels wide open, enabling the heart to supply hardworking muscles. The intelligent heart chooses the appropriate, specific genetic program, based on levels of tissue oxygenation and the energy requests of the major organs. The heart can either utilize foetal metabolism (deriving energy mostly from sugar)or it can switch to adult metabolism, which is mostly based on burning fats.

The gene that the heart activates in order to switch from one metabolism type to the other is called the peroxisome proliferator-activated receptor gamma (PPARγ). It is a gene that instantly adapts our heart to burn sugar or fat in accordance with the level of oxygen at body's disposal. The author together with Angela Rudhart-Dyczynski and Ina Sleptsova-Freidrich from Edith Cowan University, Perth in Australia had published a paper on the topic of stress and positive modulation of the genes in the Abstract book of the World Acupuncture & Integrative Medicine Conference in Houston, Texas USA in November 2014.

9. The Quantum Body and the Quantum Heart

There are multiple factors that regulate the human body. Medical physics and the laws of the fabric of the Universe both impact our health. The body reacts to different interventions in accordance with the principles of both 3D space time and medical physics, which accounts for the body's great plasticity.

Of course, everyone would like to get their body into perfect shape and maintain it in a state of a perfect health. One major priority in achieving glowing health is regular, preferably daily, exercise and respiratory muscle training. Human bodies need to walk, to run, to perform cardio exercise and to attend yoga or qi-gong classes regularly. This is news to no-one, but you really have to pay attention and actually do it. Regular physical exercise and diaphragmatic breathing training will become mapped in the brain and mind.

Sometime it's good to keep it simple. Use stairs, if it is safe, instead of the elevator. This is one of the well-known sayings of Bruce Lee, one of the most famous kung-fu fighters of the 20th century. Persevering with your exercise program will result in good physical fitness in only of three months.

To shape your physical body, you need a singular focus. Dithering and prevaricating will produce nothing but failure.

Perseverance and vigorous smart training will remodel your heart and re-shape your body. Observe your incremental progress by tracking your performance. The careful observation of changes will surprise you, and will allow you to quantify your progress. But even your best intentions may be not enough for you to reach the ultimate goal. You might need more support to boost motivation. It helps to find a friend or a professional trainer and to exercises together. Join a group or class at the gym and stick with it. The heart enjoys smart training and you will soon see big changes. Not only will your muscles, bones and tendons get stronger and more flexible, but your mind will develop resilience.

After three months of consistent, smart training you will be surprised by your new shape. New, positive feelings about your own changed body will make you feel ready for a championship.

It helps if you produce beneficial analogue waves by singing or listening to the sounds of music and nature. Enjoy one or two glasses of fresh pressed pineapple juice enriched with the pressed lemon.

Healthy nutrition can accelerate the process of remodelling the body. The knowledgeable QO will regularly consult others who are suitably skilled – a professional Quantum Observer, a personal trainer, a trusted GP, a specialist in sport medicine, a cardiologist, an acupuncturist, a massage therapist or a reflexologist – to monitor their progress and get the necessary feedback.

Even a skilled QO can sometimes have only 10 seconds to make a correct decision about their health. It could be a food choice or the selection of a place to stay. It does not really matter if the decision concerns a piece of cake or a million dollar deal. Sometimes, the QO has to decide in 10 seconds to drop an old, unhealthy friendship. In the case of the cake, for example, if you make the choice to not eat it within 10 seconds, the temptation will vanish.

During the process of intense, smart physical activity you should observe your body, and especially focus on the remodelling of the quantum heart. Listen to the messages of the heart and carefully observe the reactions to the heart's remodelling and the re-shaping of the body. The knowledgeable QO is already more sensitized to the subtle language of the heart; they still must observe the integrity of the chest and notice any irregular or disturbed heart rhythm. Watch for these symptoms:

- muscular tension or ache along arms, in the chest itself or between the shoulders
- temporary numbness in the fingers
- pain or tightness in the jaw
- a burning feeling above the stomach region can come from the overstimulated heart
- heaviness in the upper limbs
- pale face or slightly blue coloured face with stagnated blood
- tiredness
- confusion
- disorientation
- low or high blood pressure
- shortness of breath (SOB)
- agitation
- excessive sweating
- tendency to faint

These are all early Cardio symptoms and important signs. If you experience any of these symptoms while exercising, stop and perform deep abdominal breathing. And do follow up and share the symptoms with your GP or other allied health professional.

Sometimes, despite encouraging experiences with natural therapies, it is necessary to take a small dose of water soluble aspirin, or a pain killer or high dosage of vitamin C. This "self-medication" is available over-the-counter and can help to prevent some unwanted events or to get relief from distressing symptoms. However, before self-medicating, we need to read the label and understand possible side- or adverse effects. It is wise to ask a medical professional and discuss the risks of the intended self-medication.

With a transformed body shape and a positively remodelled heart, the QO will enjoy far greater vitality. The quantum body knows how to heal; it can overcome a quantum illness and it can find the open door to holistic health.

The trained QO is now skilled in the ways of achieving a positive training outcome. The knowledgeable QO has at their disposal all relevant information in their newly coded DNA by means of epigenetics, and this information can be used any time the QO wants to. Every single training unit will produce a special protein (histone) which associates with the DNA and allows new epigenetic regulations.

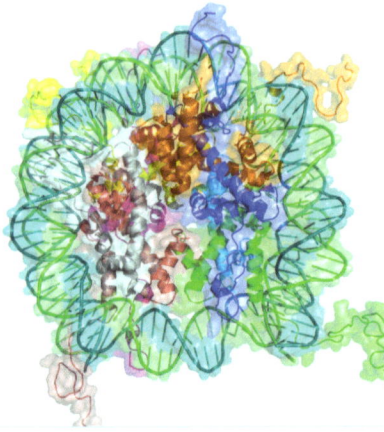

Figure 112 DNA interacting with special
histone proteins to allow epigenetic
modifications
Wikipedia Commons by Zephyris

During months of intense training you will activate healthy information and create new sequences of coding DNA. Your DNA has followed the training programme; the genes have evolved and increased their expression in order to cure the quantum heart and the quantum body. Your genes are the wise leaders guiding you in the direction of holistic healing. You should support your living DNA often, through visual feedback, acknowledgements of progress in words and in conversation with others. These activities will result in sensitive assessments and self-organizing and healing in the quantum body.

During your period of smart training, improved oxygenation will result in better bodily performance, intellectual wellness and the development of a new awareness of the body and it will lead to an expansion of consciousness.

10. Traditional Chinese Medicine and Quantum Physics

Traditional Chinese medicine is holistic. It states that the heart is the emperor, the major source of human health. Within the heart is a spirit called *Shen*, which is the source of conscience.

Shen, the Spirit in the Heart

Shen is the origin of all creative activities. Shen helps the Quantum Observer to access the invisible probability waves at the heart of the fabric of the Universe. It shapes our general health according to our intentional actions and manifests the results in the 3-D space-time world.

Shen is the major active component of the quantum heart, known in arts and literature as the metaphysical heart. Through our intentions shen manifests in the vital activities of the physical body but also explores the invisible electromagnetic dimension accessible only to human conscience.

Shen allows us to enjoy blue skies, the stars and orbiting satellites. It is holistic and not only focused on one part of human existence, on the worldly environment or on the inherited junk DNA related emotions. Shen draws our attention to the divine and to universal wisdom. It supports sublime virtues such as love, righteousness, honesty, respect and integrity. It helps to maintain the calm, wellness and the health of the whole human being. It discerns between right and wrong and evaluates the justice of actions.

Yin and Yang Building the Universe

More the 2,000 years ago traditional Chinese medicine developed a dualist view of the universe which is analogous to the quantum reality of entanglement.

The terms yin and yang are well described in the *Book of Changes*, written 221 years before Christ. It states, "Yin and yang reflect all the forms and characteristics existing in the universe". The dual aspect of the universe expresses the total relativity and the opposite qualities of yin and yang. Chapter 5 of the ancient book, entitled "Plain Questions", states, "Water and fire are the symbols for yin and yang," and this became a cornerstone of traditional Chinese medicine.

Yin and Yang and Medical Physics

The yin/yang duality of the universe is not absolute but relative. This relativity is reflected in three ways.

1. Any part of yin or yang may be indefinitely divided. Quantum physics knows the indefinite divisions that are possible to sub-particles and probability waves; they can be subdivided all the way down to superstrings and beyond

2. The interdependence of yin and yang is related to their opposite qualities, they are charged opposite to each other and yet, at the same time, they have a mutually dependent relationship. Neither can exist alone, in isolation: without yin there can be no yang, and without yang no yin. And here is the connection to quantum entanglement, to quantum health and to quantum illness

3. Yin and yang are in a relative balance. If one of them becomes dominant, it will lead to disturbance or illness. Restoring the relative balance between yin and yang is the major component of the unified probability wave and can lead to healing

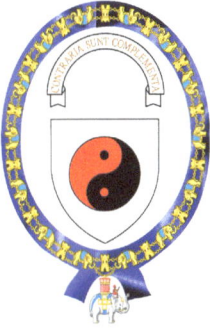

Figure 113 Niels
Bohr's coat of arms
1947
*Wiki Commons by
GJo*

The famous quantum physicist Niels Bohr found great inspiration in traditional Chinese Medicine and Chinese philosophy. He was one of the discoverers of quantum reality and he developed a new quantum model of the atom. In 1947 Bohr was knighted in recognition of his achievements for quantum physics. During this ceremony, only reserved for royals, he was dressed in a self-designed coat. His coat had arms which were featured with the traditional symbol of yin and yang and underneath had a motto in Latin: *contraria sunt complementa,* "Opposites are complementary". This red/black diagram is the Chinese symbol for the yin and yang view of the universe. It is the universal symbol of dependent opposites existing in harmony. This symbol is used in traditional Chinese medicine to signify holistic diagnostic and therapy.

Another famous quantum physicist, Fridjof Capra, was the first to bring quantum physics to public attention and he connected it to both modern and traditional Chinese medicine. Capra built a bridge between quantum physics and the eastern philosophy of Taoism. He published his bestselling book *The Tao of Physics* in 1975. Professor Capra performed experiments in quantum physics at the University of Paris, Stanford Acceleration Centre, Lawrence Berkeley Laboratory USA, Imperial College, London from 1966 to 1975.

Medical physics and traditional Chinese medicine are allied, synergistic and beneficial in common action. The alliance of both can bring great benefits to every patient. The combination of modern medical physics and traditional Chinese medicine is extremely useful in all medical situations, even under the most difficult and challenging circumstances.

11. *Respiratory Muscle Training (RMT)*

RMT and The Fundamental Meaning of Sufficient Oxygenation of the Body

Breathing is a fundamental process in sustaining your body. Pulmonology is the discipline of modern medicine covering lung function and illnesses, and the exchange of oxygen and carbon dioxide.

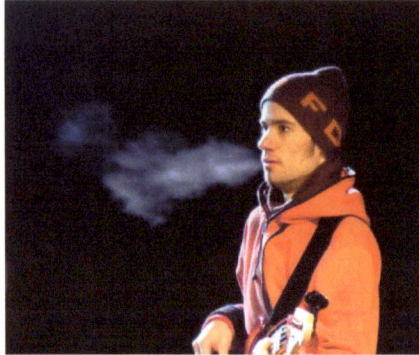

Figure 114 Visualization of the breath during exhalation in cold environment
Wikipedia Commons by Derzsi Elekes Andor

Breatheology is a science that studies how the breathing mechanism and respiratory muscle function affect longevity. Stig Severinsen, a Danish free diver is one of the most known professional sport athlete, who wrote the book in 2010- *Breathology- The Art of conscious breathing*. en.wikipedia.org/wiki/Stig Severinsen

Deep diaphragmatic breathing and strong, properly functioning respiratory muscles have a significant impact on the cardiovascular system, longevity and wellbeing. The origins of breatheology date back more than 3,000 years.

Ancient and modern scientists have been very interested in breathing techniques and respiratory muscle training. The breathing mechanism is unlike any other internal organ functions. It performs its actions independent of the mind but it can be voluntarily regulated on demand. It is well established that an improvement in breathing leads to increased energy and better health.

Contemporary breathing research takes inspiration from Indian yoga, Chinese qi-gong and Pilates. Properly conducted respiratory muscle training (RMT) can be an effective medical intervention.

3 cornerstones of breathing techniques

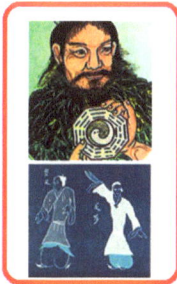

Warring States period in China
475 to 221 (before Christ) BC

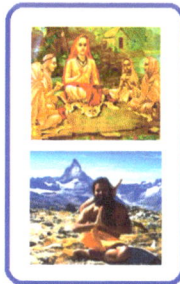

Indian scripture in sanskrit: Bhagavad Gita
between 500 and 200 before Christ BC

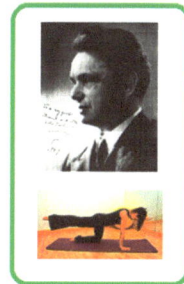

20 century Joseph H. Pilates

"Take a deep breath and make it go down to the Dan Tien. Hold it there for a while, and then breathe out the way grass germinates, until it goes up to the tip of your head. This way, your vital energy will go up, while yin goes down. The ones whose vital yin/yang energies follow their own path, shall live. The others will die"

Pranayama is the practice of the breath control. Furthermore, pranayama used in yoga means the regulation of breathing mechanism through specific breathing techniques and exercises. The sanskrit word pranayama can be translated as: "extension and control of the breath and vital life force ".

Contrology" was Joseph Pilates' preferred name for his method. Pilates targets the "modern" life-style, bad posture, and inefficient breathing as a cause for poor health. Joseph Pilates developed a series of exercises and training-techniques and engineered all the equipment. Pilate's exercises teach awareness of breath and of alignment of the spine, and strengthen the deep torso and abdominal muscles.

Figure 115 Three cornerstones of the breathing techniques: qi-gong, yoga and Pilates
Own work

High stress has an impact on the breathing mechanism and can cause shallow breathing with insufficient intake of breath. The reduced intake of air and consequent low oxygenation of the blood can directly affect brain functions, and cause low level performance across all important bodily functions.

The health of the cardiovascular system depends on the efficiency of the respiratory system. Living in an oxygen-rich environment and having an oxygen-based metabolism means that humans must use the diaphragm, chest and lungs with constant muscular force.

RMT research in 20th century focused on lung function

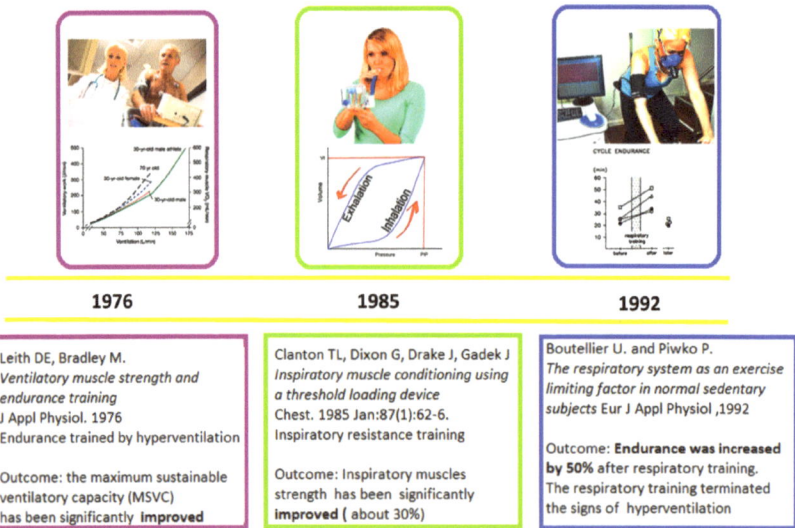

1976	1985	1992
Leith DE, Bradley M. *Ventilatory muscle strength and endurance training* J Appl Physiol. 1976 Endurance trained by hyperventilation Outcome: the maximum sustainable ventilatory capacity (MSVC) has been significantly **improved**	Clanton TL, Dixon G, Drake J, Gadek J *Inspiratory muscle conditioning using a threshold loading device* Chest. 1985 Jan:87(1):62-6. Inspiratory resistance training Outcome: Inspiratory muscles strength has been significantly **improved** (about 30%)	Boutellier U. and Piwko P. *The respiratory system as an exercise limiting factor in normal sedentary subjects* Eur J Appl Physiol ,1992 Outcome: **Endurance was increased by 50%** after respiratory training. The respiratory training terminated the signs of hyperventilation

Figure 116 The research on breathing focused in 20 century on the lung function
Own work

Modern research into respiratory muscle training (RMT) began in the 1970s. Research was focused on the lungs and the function of breathing muscles performed by Leith D.E. at al. It became clear that respiratory muscle strength or endurance can be significantly improved by specific RMT training.

A 1985 study made by Clanton T.L. at al. applied dynamic respiratory resistance breathing, using a special respiratory device that increased resistance while taking a deep breath. The results showed significant increase in inspiratory muscle strength after this kind of respiratory muscle training. The improvements came about by inducing an increased breathing rate.

In 1992, a Swiss team led by Boutellier used an RMT program to terminate hyperventilation. Boutellier and Piwko showed that respiratory endurance was increased by 50% after respiratory muscle training and that hyperventilation can be resolved after just a few RMT sessions.

The majority of studies involving lung function and respiratory muscle workout have shown that increased frequency and volume intake improves endurance and respiratory capacity. These improvements were independent of age, gender and the level of training already attained. No matter, young or old, female or male, athlete or sedentary individual, in all examined patients the lung and muscle function showed significant benefit.

Respiratory Muscle Training RMT research in the 21th century focuses on heart functions

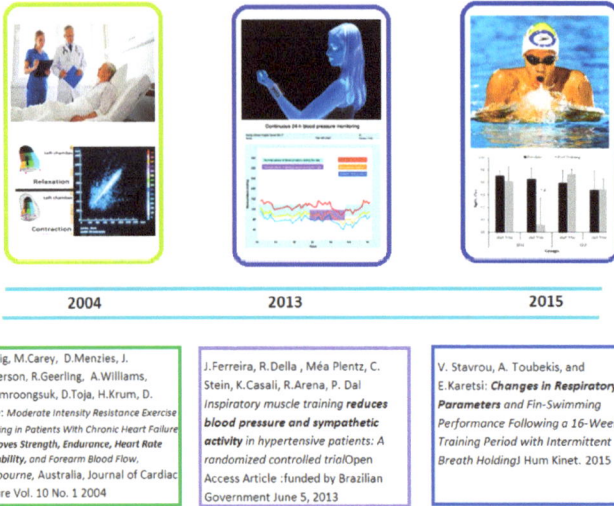

| 2004 | 2013 | 2015 |

S.Selig, M.Carey, D.Menzies, J. Patterson, R.Geerling, A.Williams, V.Bamroongsuk, D.Toja, H.Krum, D. Hare: *Moderate Intensity Resistance Exercise Training in Patients With Chronic Heart Failure Improves Strength, Endurance, Heart Rate Variability, and Forearm Blood Flow.* Melbourne, Australia, Journal of Cardiac Failure Vol. 10 No. 1 2004

J.Ferreira, R.Della , Méa Plentz, C. Stein, K.Casali, R.Arena, P. Dal *inspiratory muscle training reduces blood pressure and sympathetic activity* in hypertensive patients: A randomized controlled trialOpen Access Article :funded by Brazilian Government June 5, 2013

V. Stavrou, A. Toubekis, and E.Karetsi: *Changes in Respiratory Parameters* and Fin-Swimming Performance Following a 16-Week Training Period with Intermittent Breath HoldingJ Hum Kinet. 2015

Figure 117 The research on breathing focused in 21 century additionally to the lung function includes the intelligent heart functions
Own work

The unique manner of an individual's breathing is governed by the functions of the heart. There is a smart link between heartbeat, heart rate variability (HRV) and breathing, which was identified in 2016 and demonstrated by some Indian yogis have in a series of scientific studies made by Wenger in 1961.

A healthy heart and respiratory system enable unrestricted mobility on demand. The contracting power of the heart muscle, the independent heart beat and day/night adapted, circadian HRV each respond immediately to bodily demands. Those demands have nearly infinite variability profiles, but we each develop a number of behaviours in response to interactions between the cardiovascular system, the brain and the respiratory system. Additionally, HRV follows a circadian rhythm as the research made by Sammito S. at al confirmed in 2016. It has one pattern during the day and a very different pattern in the night.

The baseline breathing pattern of an average person can be completely controlled by the mind. Everybody can train their breathing. Then, the advanced breathing pattern can be new habituated, under one's epigenetic genetic control.

In contrast to our breathing mechanism, the heart and cardiovascular dynamics cannot be so easily controlled by the mind. The cardiovascular system operates independently, regulated by the metabolism, and the autonomic nervous system. To gain control over the cardiovascular system requires perseverance and hard training over many years.

Modern respiratory muscle training focuses on changes in heart rate variability, which provides insight into the interactions between our cardiovascular, hormonal and respiratory systems.

The breathing pattern has a genuine baseline, supplying the minimal, needed air to maintain respiration, circulation, and other vital body functions at rest. This baseline is said to be 1 MET. This basal metabolic rate accelerates during physical exercises and can reach 10 METs or even more. The respiration occurring at rest in a sitting position can be measured in litres of atmospheric air per minute and an average person has the volume about 6 litres. This is called the basal respiration rate defined by Duffin at all. in 2014. Respiration can increase 10 fold to 60 litres per minute.

The metabolic use of oxygen (O^2) and the production of carbon dioxide (CO^2) are increased during exercise, stress and other emotional reactions. An accelerated metabolism consumes more oxygen and causes the overproduction of metabolic wastes decreasing the pH of the blood, causing it to acidify. In turn the acidic pH stimulates the respiratory centre to pace breathing with the aim to remove the CO2 and to reduce acidity.

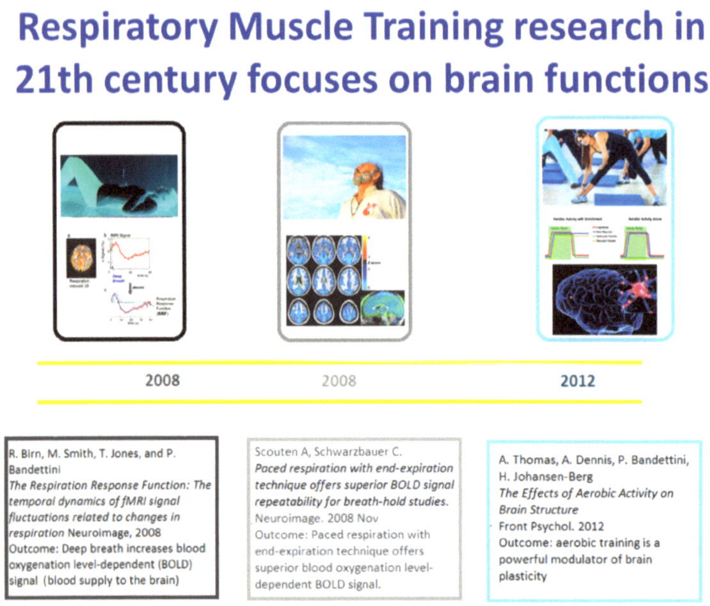

Respiratory Muscle Training research in 21th century focuses on brain functions

| 2008 | 2008 | 2012 |

| R. Birn, M. Smith, T. Jones, and P. Bandettini *The Respiration Response Function: The temporal dynamics of fMRI signal fluctuations related to changes in respiration* Neuroimage, 2008 Outcome: Deep breath increases blood oxygenation level-dependent (BOLD) signal (blood supply to the brain) | Scouten A, Schwarzbauer C. *Paced respiration with end-expiration technique offers superior BOLD signal repeatability for breath-hold studies.* Neuroimage. 2008 Nov Outcome: Paced respiration with end-expiration technique offers superior blood oxygenation level-dependent BOLD signal. | A. Thomas, A. Dennis, P. Bandettini, H. Johansen-Berg *The Effects of Aerobic Activity on Brain Structure* Front Psychol. 2012 Outcome: aerobic training is a powerful modulator of brain plasticity |

Figure 118 Respiratory Muscle Training research in 21th century focuses additionally on brain functions
Own work

Hypoxia is a state of low oxygenation of the body's tissues and internal organs and can be caused by chronic shallow breathing. Particularly it puts the brain at risk. The research on respiratory muscle training includes also its effects on the brain functionality in the 21st century .

A 2017 study performed by Dr Lawley JS and his team demonstrated that a significant decline of the brain's baseline occurred after just 2 hours of hypoxia. This was a breakthrough study in research for RMT. The summary of this breakthrough study is displayed below.

Paradigm Shift study on brain performance and hypoxia 2017

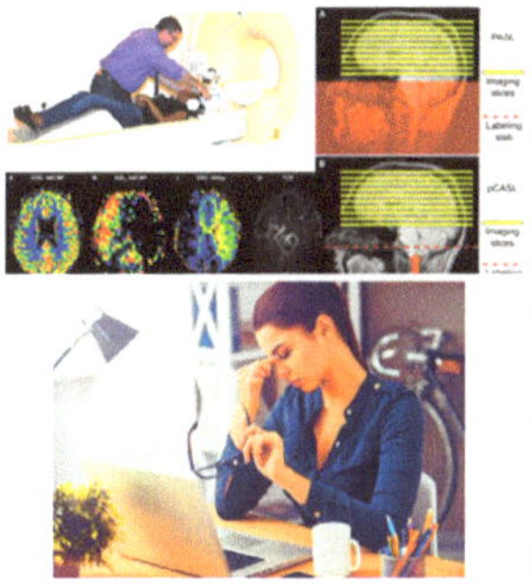

Lawley JS, Macdonald JH Oliver SJ· Mullins PG
Unexpected reductions in regional cerebral perfusion during prolonged hypoxia.
J Physiol. 2017 Feb
Outcome: **The results showed that hypoxia in brain's default mode network (DMN) can cause previously reported deficits in cognitive performance and deficits in working memory**

- Cognitive performance is impaired by hypoxia despite global cerebral oxygen delivery and metabolism being maintained

- Using arterial spin labelled (ASL) magnetic resonance imaging, this is the first study to show regional reductions in cerebral blood flow (CBF) in response to decreased oxygen supply (hypoxia) at 2 h that increased in area and became more pronounced at 10 h

- Reductions in cerebral Blood flow (CBF)were seen in brain regions typically associated with the 'default mode'

- Regional reductions in CBF, and associated vasoconstriction, within the default mode network in hypoxia

- These results suggest an anatomical mechanism through which hypoxia may cause pr eviously reported deficits in cognitive performance and cause deficits in working memory

Figure 119 A summary of the breakthrough study on low oxygenation of the brain - hypoxia
Own work

The brain's baseline, known as the default mode network (DMN), is highly sensitive to lack of oxygen (hypoxia), which threatens the core of our personality and can cause memory loss. Reduced DMN activity and low heart rate variability HRV has been found in dementia. More than 50 million people worldwide experience diverse forms of dementia now. It is critically important that the brain and its DMN maintain a good supply of oxygen-rich blood. You can support your brain's oxygen supply by focusing on the internal functions of the body including its respiratory system. Engage in deep concentration during prayer or meditation, perform regular breathing exercises.

The HRV day/night rhythm evident from study made by Sammito S. at al. was subject to a systematic research review. It has focused of 12 randomized studies performed on respiratory muscle training. They found that respiratory muscle training improves aerobic (oxygen dependent) capacity in heart failure. The authors observed an improvement of the essential cardiovascular parameters such as: cardiac volumes, skeletal muscle function, peripheral blood flow and blood vessel function. Another research group led by Lin S.J also found that RMT improves respiratory muscle strength, functional capacity, and reliefs the shortness of breath.

Heart conditions are not rare exceptions in western population. On the contrary, almost everybody has a functional or structural heart condition, an imperfection in the quantum heart or even a manifested heart condition.

A very interesting study confirming the benefits of controlled breathing and the negative effects of high stress on HRV and respiratory workout had been performed by Bernardi L. and other researchers from the Department of Internal Medicine, IRCCS S. Matteo-University of Pavia, Italy. Another study performed in 2000 showed that controlled breathing increases respiration while distress reduces it. In particular, the authors observed that as mental distress increases, breathing become shallower.

The most effective method for delivering increased oxygen to te cells and stimulating a balance bodily energy is the use the diaphragmatic breathing.

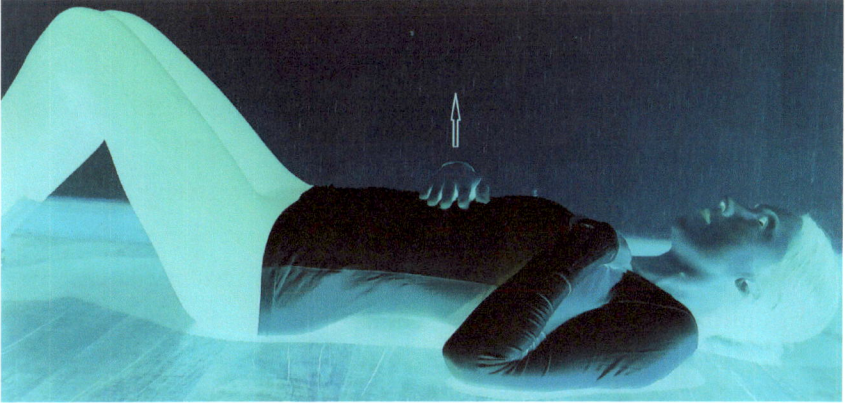

Figure 120 Diaphragmatic breathing in lying position
Courtesy Brittany Ford. Brittany is excellent in effective breathing
technics for Cardiovascular system and a remarkable nutritionist

Here's how:

1. Lie down somewhere comfortable
2. Inhale – fill the lower part of your abdomen by diaphragmatic inhalation
3. Keep inhaling – expand the middle section of chest, increasing volume
4. Even more – fill the upper chest and the top of the lungs, just below the collar bones to the brim
5. Hold for 3 – 7 seconds for increased oxygen ingestion. This will maximise gas exchange in the lungs
6. Then exhale, forcefully and completely, with a big "whoosh"

Do this 5 to 10 times. It does not take long before you feel refreshed and energized. Watch for any change in your brain, such as light-headedness or dizziness. Some people experience joy and laugh uncontrollably. This is a positive reaction, indicating increased blood supply and oxygen to brain.

With this this simple breathing technique, you can have recycled stress hormones, what in turn is keeping longer the heart hormones multidimensional health protection .

Further Reading about RMT

1. Choi J, Gutierrez-Osuna R. "Removal of respiratory influences from heart rate variability in stress monitoring". *IEEE Sensors J.* 2011; 11:2649–2656

2. Leith DE, Bradley M. "Ventilatory muscle strength and endurance training" *J Appl Physiol.* 1976

3. Boutellier U. and Piwko P. "The respiratory system as an exercise limiting factor in normal sedentary subjects", *Eur J Appl Physiol* ,1992

4. Clanton TL, Dixon G, Drake J, Gadek JE. "Inspiratory muscle conditioning using a threshold loading device". *Chest,* 1985 Jan;87(1):62-6.

5. Duffin J. "The fast exercise drive to breathe" *J Physiol.* 2014 Feb 1; 592 https://www.ncbi.nlm.nih.gov/pmc/articles/PMC393043

6. Suh-Jen L., Jessica McElfresh,, Benjamin Hall, Rachel Bloom and Kellie Farrell "Inspiratory Muscle Training in Patients with Heart Failure. A Systematic Review" Br J Sports Med. 2007 July 41(7) 407–408

7. Bernardi L., Wdowczyk-Szulc J., Valenti C., Castoldi S., Passino C. Spadacini G. "Effects of controlled breathing, mental activity and mental stress with or without verbalization on heart rate variability", *Journal of the American College of Cardiology* Volume 35, Issue 6, May 2000, Pages 1462-1469

8. Tomislav Stankovski, William H. Cooke, László Rudas, Aneta Stefanovska, Dwain L. Eckberg "Time-frequency methods and voluntary ramped-frequency breathing: a powerful combination for exploration of human neurophysiological mechanisms". *J Appl Physiol*, 2013 Dec 15; 115(12): 1806–1821.

12. Coffee in a healthy Lifestyle and Nutrition

Caffeine Blocks Adenosine and Slows Down the CLOCK Gene in the Brain

Caffeine neutralizes the calming effects of adenosine on the brain by occupying the adenosine receptors. As a result the increasing amount of adenosine in the system does not relax the brain. The brain stays alert and stimulated. The molecules of Caffeine and Adenosine are very similar.

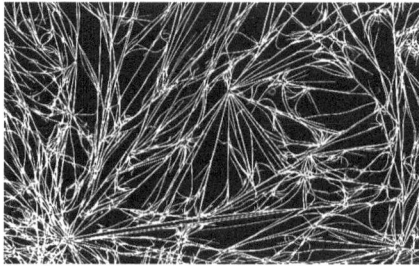

Figure 121 Caffeine crystals
Wikipedia Commons by No machine-readable author provided

From the perspective of health there are two kinds of coffee beans. Arabica beans originate from Africa and they are ground to the finest coffee with almost no gastrointestinal side effects. The growth and cultivation of Arabica is more expensive than the second type of the coffee beans, known as Robusta. Robusta beans are easier to care for and have a greater crop yield than Arabica, so at the end it is cheaper to produce, but can mighty upset our stomach.

A cup of coffee is a life style element, a pleasure and a good agent for our health. This statement is only true when the consumption of coffee is connected to a healthy lifestyle. The drinking of coffee in a nice café, accompanied by friendly conversation, or a review of newspapers and journals is different from a cup of coffee drunk in a desperate search for energy. The latter can turn into addictive self-medication.

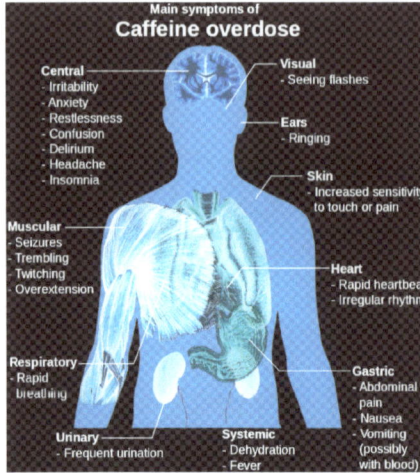

Figure 122 Caffeine overdose
Wikipedia Commons by Mikael Häggström

The origin of the coffee is Ethiopia. It produces one of the best Arabica coffees in the world.

Cafés and coffee consumption are growing, all over the world. The total consumption of both kinds of coffee amounts to over 10 million tonnes per year. Robusta is actually mostly grown in Brazil, Indonesia, India and Vietnam.

The recent development of coffee consumption has to do with its interactions with adenosine. Caffeine keeps your brain awake. We feel stronger mentally and intellectually with one or two cups of coffee. Scientific studies have confirmed that moderate caffeine consumption can have a protective effect against the development of neurodegenerative brain diseases, including Alzheimer's. The excessive consumption of Coffee as an energy drink can lead to signs of intoxication.

13. Visual Biofeedback

Something essential happens to the body when a Quantum Observer is in charge and recognizes and memorizes the visualized parameters related to their body. Blood pressure measurement is good example of the biofeedback that can enable the QO. A BP monitor displays information about the internal functioning of the body. Changes in BP are signals for the mind and the DNA to initiate a necessary change.

A smart Quantum Observer understands that the heart and cardiovascular system increase BP when there is poor oxygenation of internal organs and insufficient oxygen supply.

With some practice, you can lower your blood pressure with a few minutes of forced diaphragmatic breathing:

Take a resting position and increase the volume of your breathing using the diaphragm.

After a few minutes, repeat the blood pressure measurement and you will likely find that the action has lowered your blood pressure.

In 2011 Professor Jane Lemaire and her team from the Department of Medicine, University of Calgary in Canada published an interesting study. Their paper entitled "The Effect of a Biofeedback Based Stress Management Tool on Physicians Stress", delivered amazing results concerning the heart's response to biofeedback and confirmed the positive influence of the heart's intelligence.

Another major 2011 study showed that when a subject is given access to real time, visual feedback they experience a normalization of cardiovascular functions. After some time of observing their own ECG, the study subjects significantly lowered their stress levels and experienced more positive feelings. The beneficial results were seen in the subjects' measured health parameters such as blood pressure, heart rate, muscle tension and rhythmic breathing.

A Note on Covid-19

In the era of coronavirus pandemic your heart's health is more important than ever. Jennifer Abbasi published an article in the *Journal of the American Medical Association* (JAMA) in 2021: *Researchers Investigate what COVID-19 Does to the Heart*". It is an overview study which summarises the impact of Coronavirus infection on the heart, published very recently.

The hallmark of COVID-19 is respiratory involvement; however, severe COVID-19 has been complicated with pericardium and heart involvement. Inflammation of heart muscle (myocarditis) and the inflammatory response of the bag surrounding the heart (Pericardium) causing pericarditis are reported from hospitals all over the world.

Moreover, Covid19 related cardiac damage causes increased in-hospital mortality in COVID-19 patients who present a wide spectrum of cardiovascular symptoms, including heart failure, arrhythmias, acute coronary syndrome, myocarditis and cardiac arrest. A scientific study of a large group of **718,365** patients was published in November 2021 in the *European Journal of Medical Investigation* by Benjamin JR Buckley and his team: "Prevalence and clinical outcomes of myocarditis and pericarditis in 718,365 COVID-19 patients." published in *European Journal of Clinical Investigation*, September 2021. Heart health seems to be a crucial vital factor in surviving Covid-19. The intelligence of our heart can defend us against Coronavirus despite the fact that the virus is in constant motion because the heart never sleeps; it is a divine source of natural vitality.

When we care about the heart's electromagnetic functions it will connect us with the probability waves of the fabric of Universe. The heart will adapt us to physical influences and biological influences. Our heart buffers not only gravity and the climate, but also constant attacks by viruses and bacteria.

The pericardium is a part of lymphatic system and is primarily involved in the response to any viral infection, including Coronavirus. The direct affected pericardium and heart muscle also suffer from lack of oxygen caused by viral lung infection.

When attacked by a virus, the body undergoes stress and releases a surge of chemicals called catecholamines (stress hormones) that can stun the heart. This amounts to a three-fold attack on the heart:

1. A direct attack on the heart cells,
2. A reduction in oxygen due to lung invasion, and
3. The weakening of the heart muscle caused by overstimulation via stress hormones.

These threats to the heart are explained in detail in an article by Dr Erin Donelly Michos of John Hopkins University entitled "Can Coronavirus Cause Heart Damage?" which was publisshed in April 2020. https://www.hopkinsmedicine.org/health/conditions-and-diseases/coronavirus/can-coronavirus-cause-heart-damage

It is good to keep in mind that in 2015 the Nobel Prize went to scientists who contributed to the development of two drugs against parasites. Professor William C. Campbell and Satoshi Ōmura discovered of Ivermectin, and Dr Tu Youyou was awarded for the discovery of Artemisin. Both drugs are anti-parasitic drugs and both can potentially be effective against viruses, which are the smallest parasites.https://www.nobelprize.org/prizes/medicine/2015/press-release/

Conclusion

Your all-knowing heart's intelligence supports healing and perpetual regeneration. The intelligent heart executes its intelligence in coordinating body functions through the production and release of its own four hormones.

The intelligent heart has a much greater impact on our health, information processing and perceptions than we previously understood.

The heart's wisdom incudes the all features of the intelligent heart and, above it, a lifestyle which is accords with the laws of Universe, with the laws of quantum reality and of medical physics from the position of a Quantum Observer.

The intelligent heart loves an abundance of oxygen. Accordingly, a secret key to maintaining optimal functioning of the intelligent heart is daily RMT: Respiratory Muscle Training. When your breathing is efficient, oxygen will stream down to all of your cells and will invigorate your entire body.

The intelligent heart can protect itself in case of a shortage of oxygen by entering the hibernating myocardium state, the sleeping protective mode. In doing so it enters a state of lesser functionality but can preserve its vitality. The full understanding of the intelligent heart functions builds the foundation for good general health and for the expansion of the abundant bodily life force.

Acknowledgements

"Give thanks to the Lord for He is good, His love endures forever."
Psalms 118:29

My deepest gratitude goes to my wife Angela and my daughter Fatima. They are really co-authors of this book. My wife Angela created the term "intelligent heart" in 2009 during our scientific work at Edith Cowan University in Perth.

My gratitude goes to all of my patients for the deep medical experiences about the meaning of the heart and their mandate to share it with all for the "benefit of mankind". My daughter Fatima used that phrase in her scientific work concerning the nano-satellites delivering real time images of the Earth to everybody's mobile phone. In our conversation Fatima used to say, "The book, the book, the book..." pointing out its importance and the time factor needed for accomplish it.

The idea to write this book came directly from Marina Jankovic. Marina is a real visionary and had a glimpse of future around 2011, and saw this book about the intelligence of the heart published!

Thanks also to Laura Bond, a freelance journalist and health coach and the author of the book *Mum's Not Having Chemo*, for her suggestions about the structure of this book.

Many thanks go to Maria Bakkas-Booker and Dr Roderic Pitty for their valuable linguistic suggestions to the text of this book.

Thanks to generous Universe, and helpful colleagues and to Wikipedia and its founder Jimmy Wales, for Wiki Commons, for making available public domain and freely licensed educational media content. A big thanks to its creative authors who allowed us to use their images to illustrate this book.

Thanks from my heart to Dr. Story Musgrave, US Astronaut, student, artist, scientist, designer, engineer, mentor, educator, speaker and consultant, for permission to publish his picture of the Universe and DNA, illustrating the evolution of complexity on our planet, mother earth.

This book owes its existence Stephen Cole, the Managing Director of the eBooks.com, and his wife Trudy. Both have been pioneers of ebooks and they both gave to this book a new modern structure and the ebook spirit. They helped to render my text more accessible for the lay person. Stephen's and Trudy's eBooks.com is the only independent eBook retailer that sells into every country in the world, including Antarctica and the International Space Station!

Table of images

1. The image was created by US Astronaut Dr Story Musgrave MD, who has repaired the Hubble Telescope in space. Musgrave said, "It illustrates the evolution of complexity on our planet, mother Earth"

2. The MRI image shows two sequenced stages of the left chamber of the heart, in relaxation and contraction. LV is an abbreviation for the left ventricle (chamber). LA is left atrium. RV is the right ventricle and RA is the right atrium. Own work

3. The diagram is from "Heart Rate, Life Expectancy and the Cardiovascular System" by K. Boudoulas and his team from the Ohio State University (USA) published in the

Journal of Cardiology in 2015. https://www.karger.com/Article/FullText/435947

4. Interactions between the protective heart hormones, especially BNP, and the systemic fight-or-flight stress response, also involving adrenals and kidneys. BP stands for blood pressure, HR for heart rate and hypoxia means a substantial lack of oxygen. Own work

5. Recycling of stress hormones. Own work

6. The 7TM receptors are cell surface receptors that detect molecules and electromagnetic impulses outside the cell and activate cellular responses (Image: Wikipedia Commons Opabinia regalis - Own work, CC BY-SA 3.0)

7. An example of the mechanical wave created through the heart and registered as a pulse wave at the hand from the radial artery and at the neck from the carotid artery, own work

8. The Genetic code. Genetic code logo of the Globobulimina pseudospinescens mitochondrial genome Wikipedia Commons by Bas E. Dutilh, Rasa Jurgelenaite, Radek Szklarczyk, Sacha A.F.T. van Hijum, Harry R. Harhangi, Markus Schmid, Bart de Wild, Kees-Jan Françoijs, Hendrik G. Stunnenberg, Marc Strous, Mike S.M. Jetten, Huub J.M. Op den Camp and Martijn A. Huynen - doi: 10.1093/bioinformatics/btr316 CC BY 2.5

9. A general practitioner uses a stethoscope to listen to your heartbeat and the gentle sound of breathing Photograph author Alith3204 - Own work distributed under by Wikipedia Commons under CC BY-SA 4.0 https://en.wikipedia.org/wiki/Heart_sounds

10. Two sounds of the heart registered with microphone know as a phonocardiogram. Own work

11. An artist's vision of the electromagnetic field of the body. Own work

12. Electrocardiogram with three major waves P, QRS and T with their origins. Own work

13. Electrocardiogram (ECG) on the left side of the picture, and the magnetocardiogram MCG on the right. Own work

14. One full electrical cycle of a heartbeat. The electronic drawing of a modern registration of both an electrocardiogram ECG (bottom of the picture) and magnetocardiogram MCG (in the upper part).Own work

15. Two-dimensional space depicted in three-dimensional space-time. The past and future light cones are absolute, the "present" is a relative concept different for observers in relative motion. Photograph author K. Aainsqatsi at en.wikipedia, transferred from en.wikipedia to Commons distributed under CC BY-SA 3.0

16. The human body is holistically designed for exploring invisible electromagnetic reality, the functions of the spirit by the heart and the functioning of the awareness in the 3 D reality by the brain/mind. The duration of the individual life span displayed as the DNA line relates to the balance between operational, spiritual activity in the hidden reality of the fabric of the Universe and the actions in the solid 3D reality. Own work

17. The spirit explores the spiritual, invisible and hidden electromagnetic dimension, and builds the grid for the operations of consciousness. The strongest power is attributed to the intention. Own work

18. The supersymetry in the universe and in nature empowers our fundamental understanding of the cosmos, from the universality of gravity to the unification of the forces of nature at higher energy levels. The letter E stands for electron, P for proton. G for gravity and the related three s letters are symbolically the predicted super symmetry

particles, own work with four extracts of the images from the documentary film The Elegant Universe: Welcome to the 11th Dimension by Dr Brian Greene, an American theoretical physicist and professor at the Columbia University. https://www.youtube.com/watch?v=GdqC2bV-LesQ

19. Analogue, rhythmic cycles such as the electrocardiogram ECG are fundamental for dynamic interactions in the human body. Own work

20. The result of chronic heart failure is an enlarged heart as seen in this chest x-ray. Enlargement can also be detected by means of an ultrasound or MRI scan. Own work

21. The anatomy of the heart showing the left atrium, where the production of adult omnipotent stem cells take place. ANP stimulates the production of omnipotent stem cells and brings life-sustaining minerals, such as sodium, potassium and magnesium back into balance. Photograph by Wapcaplet -Own work distributed under Wikipedia Commons CC BY-SA 3.0

22. Atrial Natriuretic Peptide ANP granules, Photograph from the personal laboratory pictures Dr Pang, he is a researcher at Queen University in Kingston, Ontario., CC BY-SA 3.0, https://commons.wikimedia.org/w/index.php?curid=74824545

23. Displays the 3D structure of natriuretic peptide B (BNP,) with the ANP-receptor in purple color. Wikipedia, Public domain released from: X.L.He et al. Structural determinants of natriuretic peptide receptor specificity and degeneracy. J Mol Biol, 361, 698-714. PMID 16870210 [DOI: 10.1016/j.jmb.2006.06.060

24. Molecular structure of the C-Type natriuretic peptide CNP from the Department of Physiology of The Institute of Arctic Medicine at the Oulu University, Finland

25. The image of knotted DNA is credited to N. Cozzarelli. The mechanism of self-entanglement is a genetic attempt to repair the corrupted DNA

26. Transcription the information from the DNA to RNA and splicing of the genes from pre-mRNA (messenger RNA) Photograph by Ganeshmanohar - Own work, CC BY-SA 4.0 https://commons.wikimedia.org/w/index.php?curid=75544197

27. Eastern green mamba, native to the coastal regions of southern East Africa. Wikipedia by Neil - https://www.flickr.com/photos/neilhooting/3554348399/, CC BY 2.0 https://commons.wikimedia.org/w/index.php?curid=18705595)

28. The structural similarity between Caffeine and Adenosine. It is the reason why the caffeine keeps us alert and vigilant. Wikipedia Commons, No machine-readable source provided. Own work assumed (based on copyright claims) https://commons.wikimedia.org/w/index.php?curid=1073148

29. Vortex flow in all chambers of the heart captured during a MRI procedure. A turbulent flow is marked in the left ventricle (LV). Own work

30. The progression of harm that is possible in a heart attack. Own work

31. Patient with a portable oxygen concentrator. Own work

32. A blood clot. The platelets, the fibrin mesh and the immune system cells inside of a blood vessel. Blausen.com staff (2014). "Medical gallery of Blausen Medical 2014". WikiJournal of Medicine 1 (2). DOI:10.15347/wjm/2014.010. ISSN 2002-4436. Own work

33. Elly's coronary calcium scan from 2012. Her calcium score was 496 bottom part of the picture. The modern CT Coronary Angiography (CCTA) scan of Elly's heart

in 2021—a more sophisticated technique, which can visualize the white calcium spots, and the course of coronary arteries and their plaques at the upper part of the picture. Own work. Courtesy Elly W.

34. Coronary angioplasty, or percutaneous coronary intervention (PCI), is non-surgical procedure to treat narrowing of the coronary arteries with a balloon. Picture credit: https://commons.wikimedia.org/w/index.php?curid=19334307

35. The picture on the left shows a coronary artery and the magnification shows the coronary vessel with the implanted stent. By BruceBlaus. Blausen.com staff (2014). " Medical gallery of Blausen Medical 2014" WikiJournal of Medicine 1 (2). DOI:10.15347/wjm/2014.010. ISSN 2002-4436. - Own work, CC BY 3.0, https://commons.wikimedia.org/w/index.php?curid=33041225

36. A color coded MRI scan of a heart with restored coronary blood flow after a successful coronary angiography. The coronary vessels are all open and supplying the heart muscle. Own work

37. Representation of a DNA molecule that is methylated. The two white spheres represent methyl groups. A sequence of DNA. Wikipedia Commons by Christoph Bock, Max Planck Institute for Informatics - Own work, CC BY-SA 3.0 https://commons.wikimedia.org/w/index.php?curid=17066877

38. The G-Proteins are coloured red, orange and brown at the picture. They translate the impulses from the 7TM receptor outside the cell and transmit them to the cell's interior, to the DNA situated in the cell's nucleus. Courtesy Tony P.

39. The heart creates analogue frequency. It can be recorded as an ECG, showing the electrical cyclic waves originating from the heart. The black cyclic ECG complexes are normal; the red ones display abnormal heart beats. Own work

40. An EEG displays four forms of brain waves known as beta, alpha, theta and delta, which are different ranges of frequencies. Own work

41. Plaque can restrict blood flow to the heart muscle by physically clogging the artery or by causing abnormal artery tone. https://www.myupchar.com/en/disease/coronary-artery-disease, CC BY-SA 4.0

42. The blood pressure fluctuates throughout the day and night, but the average values are usually within the normal or optimal range. Own work.

43. Developing brain blood vessels, known as vasculature. The small vessels include small, reactive muscles opening wide to nerve impulses. The vessel network undergoes not only angiogenic sprouting (arrowheads white), but also extensive vessel pruning. By Sedwick C (2012) Pruning Brain Vasculature for Efficiency. PLoS Biol 10(8): e1001375. doi:10.1371/journal.pbio.1001375. This file was published in a Public Library of Science journal. Their website states that the content of all PLOS journals is published under the Creative Commons Attribution 4.0 license

44. It is common knowledge that atrial fibrillation (AF) carries a high risk of stroke. The illustration shows how a stroke can occur during atrial fibrillation. A blood clot (thrombus) can form in the left atrium of the heart. If a piece of the clot breaks off and travels to an artery in the brain, it can block blood flow through the artery. The lack of blood flow to the portion of the brain fed by the artery causes a stroke. Credit for the image is to the National

45. In a "broken heart", the left ventricle takes on the shape of a takotsubo, a Japanese trap used to catch octopi. J. Heuser CC BY-SA 3.0 <http://creativecommons.org/licenses/by-sa/3.0/>, via WikimediaCommons https://en.wikipedia.org/wiki/Takotsubo_cardiomyopathy#/media/File:TakoTsubo_scheme.png

46. Map of the electromagnetic field of the Earth, Wikipedia. https://en.wikipedia.org/wiki/File:World_Magnetic_Field_2015.pdf

47. Skin is built from powerful, resilient layers of collagen, laminin and integrin. It separates the bio-universe inside from the vast universe outside. Image: Credit to Biolamina http://www.biolamina.com/basement-membrane-proteins

48. A small portable device for registration of ECG and HRV . Own work with an extract from the Electro Heart Port, Energy-Lab Technologies, Hamburg, Germany

49. A normal distribution of three frequencies of HRV related to breathing/lung function, heart/brain interactions and hormonal/immune system activity. Own work

50. The cardio stress index (CSI), the Cardio Image on the left side was increased with 56%. The increased stress level is displayed as the brown coloration at the core, the "lead" of the Heart Image. The redness on the left could be related to a hibernation of a small heart area. On the right side of the image almost a normalization of the Cardio Image after acupuncture and respiratory muscle training

51. Twenty four hours registration of HRV. Own work

52. A section of an ECG reading with fundamental time measurements of heart rate variability HRV. It shows the small

The opening "Heart Lung and Blood Institute (NIH), Public domain, via Wikimedia Commons" appears before item 45.

but countable differences between regular heartbeats. Own work

53. Cardio Image of a patient in a moment of stress as a brown at the core of the Cardio Image and a limited HRV, a very small and short "torpedo/comet" indicated in the Poincaré-Plot diagram. Own work

54. The Cardio Image displayed above originates from the same patient .After treatment with medical acupuncture and a short respiratory muscle training the patient's profile returned to normal indicated by the green colour at the core of the Cardio Image and improved in the HRV Poincaré-Plot diagram indicated as a bigger and longer "torpedo/comet". Own work

55. Heart Cardio Images of a patient before and after treatment. The Cardio Image on the left reflects a stressful situation. Increased stress is displayed as the brown coloration at the core, the "lead" of the heart Cardio Image on the left side. The Cardio Image on the right was recorded after respiratory muscle training (RMT) and medical acupuncture, about 1 hour later. The green/blue colour of the follow up Cardio Image registration indicated the return of patient's normal profile. Own work

56. Electrical impulses are caused by calcium sparks initiating every single heartbeat. Own work

57. Registration of Cardio Image and HRV using Vicardio. Own work

58. A typical healthy pattern of an ECG reading. It shows four waves originating from the initial excitation, mechanical contraction and relaxation of the heart muscle. Own work

59. Diagram shows a complete ECG complex and the origin of the P wave- contraction of the atria, ORS complex-con-

traction of the chambers and the T wave-relaxation of the heart chambers. Own work

60. Image of a finger pulse oximeter. The bigger number 94 indicates the oxygen blood saturation and 77 is the pulse rate. Own work

61. The quantum probability approach is at least as important in medicine and in our daily lives as the four forces of nature set out in fundamental physics: electromagnetic field, gravitation, weak interaction between particles and atomic strong interaction. Own work

62. The path of the electron beam is curved in a magnetic field. Cathode Ray Tube by Pseudo1 Intellectual

63. Niels Bohr's quantum model of an atom with electrons changing their orbits, and emitting quanta of light modified. Created by JabberWok, the Bohr model Wiki Commons CC BY-SA 3.0. https://en.wikipedia.org/wiki/Bohr_model#/media/File:Bohr_atom_model.svg

64. Artist's impression of a black hole system. Image Credit: Dana Berry, NASA

65. Probability waves of the fabric of the Universe and the equation describing it. It is credited to video quantum world and reality, World Science Festival https://www.youtube.com/watch?v=GdqC2bVLesQ

66. Superstrings of the fabric of the Universe. This image is credited to video quantum world and reality, World Science Festival. https://www.youtube.com/watch?v=GdqC2bVLesQ

67. Timeline of the universe. In this diagram, time passes from left to right, so at any given time, the universe is represented by a disk-shaped "slice" of the diagram. Picture credited to NASA. http://pics-about-space.com/end-of-the-universe-nasa?p=4# By NASA/WMAP Science Team - Original version: NASA; modified by Cherkash, Public

Domain, https://commons.wikimedia.org/w/index.php?curid=11885244

68. Modern MRI scanner and the MRI scanner gradient magnets. Image credited to Amber Diagnostics. https://www.amberusa.com/blog/gradient-coils-inside-mri-what-you-need-to-know/

69. Hydrogen atom. Extract from the image by Bruce Blaus Blausen.com staff (2014). "Medical gallery of Blausen Medical 2014". WikiJournal of Medicine 1 (2). DOI:10.15347/wjm/2014.010. ISSN 2002-4436.Wikipedia Commons

70. The quark structure of the proton. Created by Arpad Horvath – Wikipedia Commons CC BY-SA 2.5 https://en.wikipedia.org/wiki/Proton#/media/File:Quark_structure_proton.svg

71. Random directed Hydrogen protons are aligned in one direction during a Magnetic Resonance Imaging MRI. Berger A. Magnetic resonance imaging. Own work with reference to: BMJ. 2002;324(7328):35. doi:10.1136/bmj.324.7328.35

72. Colour coded visualization of MRI of the brain. Wikipedia Commons, by © Nevit Dilmen, CC BY-SA 3.0, https://commons.wikimedia.org/w/index.php?curid=19929099

73. The Kármán line is beginning about 100 kilometres above the Earth. The Kármán line defines a boundary between Earth's atmosphere and outer space. Wikipedia Commons by NASA Earth Observatory http://eol.jsc.nasa.gov/scripts/sseop/photo.pl?mission=ISS013&roll=E&frame=54329, Public Domain, https://commons.wikimedia.org/w/index.php?curid=1722627

74. Artist concept of Gravity Probe B orbiting the Earth to measure space-time, a four-dimensional description of the universe including height, width, length, and time. Wikipedia Commons by NASA - http://www.nasa.gov/mission_pages/gpb/gpb_012.html, Public Domain, https://commons.wikimedia.org/w/index.php?curid=4072432

75. Interactions of organisms with electromagnetic fields from across the electromagnetic spectrum are part of bio-electromagnetic studies. Created by Inductive load, NASA - self-made, information by NASA based of File: EM Spectrum3-new by NASA The butterfly icon is from the P icon set, File:P biology.svg. The humans are from the Pioneer plaque, File:Human.svg. The buildings are the Petronas towers and the Empire State Buildings, both from File:Skyscrapercompare.svg, CC BY-SA 3.0, https://commons.wikimedia.org/w/index.php?curid=2974242

76. Quantum probability approach of a Quantum Observer QO and the intention for healing. Own work

77. Entanglement. Wikipedia Commons by JasonHise - Own work, CC0, Universal Public Domain Dedication https://commons.wikimedia.org/w/index.php?curid=37554958

78. Relation between 3D reality and the fabric of Universe with the intention of a QO. Own work with an extract from World Science Festival. https://www.youtube.com/watch?v=GdqC2bVLesQ

79. An energized electron passes through a barrier in an example of quantum tunnelling. An example of Tunnel Effect - The evolution of the wave function of an electron through a potential barrier. The original uploader was

Jean-Christophe BENOIST at French Wikipedia. - Transferred from French Wikipedia to Wikipedia Commons

80. Major medical and natural medicine disciplines building the framework of the holistic medicine. Own work

81. Relationship between 3D reality +time and the awareness and consciousness oh an individual searching for healing and own health integrity. Drawing by Angela Rudhart-Dyczynski

82. Five components of quantum Illness: 1. Traumatized Self 2. Self Satisfaction 3. Double Agenda. 4. Deal with Death. 5. Supertrauma. Own work

83. Relation between awareness, consciousness and justice in a life span of an individual. Own work

84. Acupuncture as a quantum medical intervention. The acupuncture needles interact with the human electromagnetic body field. Own work

85. The brain default mode network is made up of defined anatomical structures in the brain. The DMN is a cluster of structures in the brain that keep the core of the individual personality active. These structures conduct very dense informational traffic because they hold and maintain the core of your personality. Own work with extract from images by Andreashorn - Own work, CC BY-SA 4.0, https://commons.wikimedia.org/w/index.php?curid=34327919

86. The pathways are displaying the informational traffic in the brain. Images by Andreashorn - Own work, CC BY-SA 4.0, https://commons.wikimedia.org/w/index.php?curid=34327919

87. Acupuncture intervention to restore the normal function of the brain's default network DMN. Own work. Courtesy Joley H.

88. A patient undergoing qEEG. On the right is the 4-colour display of the EEG output. Own work

89. The cell membrane. Wikipedia Commons by LadyofHats Mariana Ruiz - Own work. Image renamed from File:.svg, Public Domain, https://commons.wikimedia.org/w/index.php?curid=6027169

90. Electromagnetic receptor in Bruce Lipton's book "The New Biology. Own work with the image of the cover of the Bruce Lipton's book "New Biology"

91. Movement of water and water soluble substances through the cell membrane. Wikipedia Commons by BruceBlau :Blausen.com staff (2014). Medical gallery of Blausen Medical 2014" WikiJournal of Medicine 1 (2). DOI:10.15347/wjm/2014.010. ISSN 2002-4436. - Own work, CC BY 3.0, https://commons.wikimedia.org/w/index.php?curid=29140354

92. The cell membrane creating the electromagnetic potential trough movements of ions of Sodium and Potassium. Wikipedia Commons by LadyofHats Mariana Ruiz Villarreal - Own work. Image renamed from Image: Sodium-Potassium.pump.svg, Public Domain, https://commons.wikimedia.org/w/index.php?curid=3981038

93. The picture displays two readings of a Cardio Images for the same patient before and after acupuncture. Note the positive change of the colours, the brown/violet coloration turned to blue/green, what is considered to be a sign of the significant reduction of the stress level. Own work

94. Electromagnetic water in the human body. Own work

95. Electromagnetic constitution of the human body. Own work

96. Electrical synapse in the human body. Wikipedia Commons by Mariana Ruiz LadyofHats - the diagram i made myself using the information on this websites as source: [1], [2], [3], and[4]. Made with Adobe Illustrator. Image renamed from File:Gap cell junction.svg, Public Domain, https://commons.wikimedia.org/w/index.php?curid=6027074

97. Artemisia Absinthium and Artemisia Annua. Artemisia annua is known for its anti-malaria and anti-viral properties. Artemisia absinthium is known as a very useful agent against parasites, and it has anti-viral activity. Wikipedia Commons by AfroBrazilian, CC BY-SA 3.0 <https://creativecommons.org/licenses/by-sa/3.0>, via Wikimedia Commons

98. Transmission the message from the electromagnetic receptor to the DNA. The message is coded through the change of the shape of the receptor. Own work

99. The picture illustrates the crystalline structure of an activated 7TM receptor (blue colour) and its interaction with a hormone marked yellow (for example Adrenaline). Picture adopted from the information for the public, Nobel Prize in Chemistry in 2012

100. The CLOCK gene. Wikipedia Commons by Ismaïl Jarmouni - Own work, CC BY-SA 4.0,

101. Downgrading of 7TM receptors. Own work. Courtesy Tony P.

102. The common localisation of heartaches. Own work

103. The author with Dr Mosley in Perth, at the medical conference Science on the Swan in 2019

104. Daughter of the author Miss Fatima Dyczynski B.Sc. Aerospace Engineer during her TEDX lecture in The Netherlands in 2013: "Make space personal" https://www.youtube.com/watch?v=CJ0WhWLXsIE

105. Classical acupuncture with cooper handled needles. Own work.

106. Acupuncture mechanical impact of the needle creates hormonal and cellular responses

107. Heart meridian with all 9 acupuncture points. The seventh acupuncture point H7 is known in Chinese language as shenmen. It means, translated to English, "the gate to the spirit". Own work

108. The image displays the localisation of the typical pain caused by angina pectoris (tightness of the chest) or a heart attack. On the right side the course of the heart meridian as it is displayed in the most books of acupuncture and traditional Chinese medicine. Own work

109. The acupuncture on the seventh point of the heart meridian H7.Own work

110. Acupuncture as a quantum medical intervention. Own work with an image from Tzou CH, Yang TY, Chung YC. Evaluation of heat transfer in acupuncture needles: convection and conduction approaches. J Acupunct Meridian Stud. 2015 Apr;8(2):77-82. doi: 10.1016/ j.jams.2014.07.001. Epub 2014 Jul 22. PMID: 25952124 https://www.sciencedirect.com/science/article/pii/ S2005290114001174?via%3Dihub

111. The image displays a 37 year old police officer who was released from his chronic headache after three medical acupuncture treatments. Please note the increase of blood supply in the skin, deep relaxation of muscles, especially the shoulder region and even more electrified hairs. Own work

112. DNA interacting with special histone proteins to allow epigenetic modifications. Wikipedia Commons by Zephyris at the English - language Wikipedia, CC BY-SA

3.0, https://commons.wikimedia.org/w/index.php?curid=6998210

113. Niels Bohr's coat of arms, 1947. Argent, a taijitu (yin-yang symbol) Gules and Sable. Motto: Contraria sunt complementa ("opposites are complementary") by GJo - Own work from File:Royal Coat of Arms of Denmark.svg (Collar of the Order of the Elephant) + File:Yin yang.svg. For images of his coat of arms as displayed at Frederiksborg Castle, Denmark, see: [1], [2], [3], CC BY-SA 3.0, https://commons.wikimedia.org/w/index.php?curid=9680951

114. Visualization of the breath during exhalation in cold environment. Wikipedia Commons by Derzsi Elekes Andor from Budapest. Visualization of the breath during exhalation in cold environment. This file is licensed under the Creative Commons Attribution-Share Alike 4.0 International https://en.wikipedia.org/wiki/Breathing#/media/File:Bak%C3%B3_%C3%81rp%C3%A1d_-_Milagro_(Santana_Tribute)_egy%C3%BCttes,_Miskolc,_2015.02.07_(8).JPG

115. Three cornerstones of the breathing techniques: qi-gong, yoga and Pilates

116. The research on breathing focused in 20 century on the lung function, own work

117. The research on breathing focused in 21 century additionally to the lung function on the intelligent heart functions

118. Respiratory Muscle Training research in 21th century focuses additionally on brain functions. Own work

119. A summary of the breakthrough study on low oxygenation of the brain – hypoxia. Own work

120. Diaphragmatic breathing in lying position. Courtesy Brittany Ford. Brittany is excellent in effective breathing technics for Cardio and a remarkable nutritionist.

https://www.facebook.com/Busy-Body-Nutri-tion-107618964818762/

121. Caffeine crystals. Wikipedia Commons by No machine-readable author provided. The author Icey assumed (based on copyright claims). - Own work assumed (based on copyright claims). Public Domain, https://commons.wiki-media.org/w/index.php?curid=1073148

122. Caffeine overdose. Wikipedia Commons by Mikael Häggström - All used images are in public domain. https://commons.wikimedia.org/w/in-dex.php?curid=6236794

About Dr Dyczynski

Dr Jerzy Dyczynski MD, MBA is a medical doctor who is passionate about both mainstream and holistic medicine. He has worked as a medical doctor and a medical acupuncturist for more than 30 years in Poland, Germany, Switzerland and Australia, in public and private health care systems.

Jerzy is a cardiologist, an internal medicine specialist and a Doctor of Medical Sciences. He has published papers in over 70 international journals and has given more than a hundred scientific presentations on the global stage.

He completed studies as an acupuncturist in Beijing from 1991 to 1997.

Dr Jerzy attained qualifications in medical quality management for physicians of the Bavarian Medical Council, Munich, between 1999 and 2000, including training: moderation, medical leadership, epidemiology, information systems, organizational techniques, quality dimensions and methods of interdisciplinary safety models, in business process management, quality management strategies, and quality and risk management.

Dr Jerzy received his doctorate in Cardiology in 2002 and graduated with a medical MBA in the management of outpatient and integrated medical care.

Since 2007 he has lived in Perth, Western Australia, where he has practiced as a rural GP and as a postgraduate researcher in heart-brain medicine. He has practiced as an acupuncturist at Edith Cowan University, as well as in private practice in Western Australia.

Jerzy has practiced Qi-gong and Kung Fu for more than 20 years and has published two books on the nexus between Eastern and Western medicine.

www.ingramcontent.com/pod-product-compliance
Lightning Source LLC
Chambersburg PA
CBHW040928030426
42334CB00002B/4